LIVING WITH FOOD ALLERGY

ALEX GAZZOLA is an author, journalist, researcher and writing tutor who has written widely on health, food and nutritional issues. He has a special interest in food sensitivities and digestion, and his previous book, *Living with Food Intolerance*, is also published by Sheldon Press. He can be contacted through his website at www.alexgazzola.co.uk

Overcoming Common Problems Series

Selected titles
A full list of titles is available from Sheldon Press,
36 Causton Street, London SW1P 4ST, and on our website at
www.sheldonpress.co.uk

Overcoming Common Problems Series

Coping with a Mid-life Crisis
Derek Milne

Coping with Polycystic Ovary Syndrome
Christine Craggs-Hinton

Coping with Postnatal Depression
Sandra L. Wheatley

Coping with SAD
Fiona Marshall and Peter Cheevers

Coping with Snoring and Sleep Apnoea
Jill Eckersley

Coping with a Stressed Nervous System
Dr Kenneth Hambly and Alice Muir

Coping with Strokes
Dr Tom Smith

Coping with Suicide
Maggie Helen

Coping with Thyroid Problems
Dr Joan Gomez

Depression
Dr Paul Hauck

Depression at Work
Vicky Maud

Depressive Illness
Dr Tim Cantopher

Eating for a Healthy Heart
Robert Povey, Jacqui Morrell and Rachel
Povey

Effortless Exercise
Dr Caroline Shreeve

Fertility
Julie Reid

Free Your Life from Fear
Jenny Hare

Getting a Good Night's Sleep
Fiona Johnston

**Heal the Hurt: How to Forgive
and Move On**
Dr Ann Macaskill

Heart Attacks – Prevent and Survive
Dr Tom Smith

Help Your Child Get Fit Not Fat
Jan Hurst and Sue Hubberstey

Helping Children Cope with Anxiety
Jill Eckersley

**Helping Children Cope with Change and
Loss**
Rosemary Wells

**Helping Children Get the Most from
School**
Sarah Lawson

How to Be Your Own Best Friend
Dr Paul Hauck

How to Beat Pain
Christine Craggs-Hinton

How to Cope with Bulimia
Dr Joan Gomez

How to Cope with Difficult People
Alan Houel and Christian Godefroy

How to Improve Your Confidence
Dr Kenneth Hambly

How to Keep Your Cholesterol in Check
Dr Robert Povey

How to Stick to a Diet
Deborah Steinberg and Dr Windy Dryden

How to Stop Worrying
Dr Frank Tallis

Hysterectomy
Suzie Hayman

Is HRT Right for You?
Dr Anne MacGregor

Letting Go of Anxiety and Depression
Dr Windy Dryden

Lifting Depression the Balanced Way
Dr Lindsay Corrie

Living with Alzheimer's Disease
Dr Tom Smith

Living with Asperger Syndrome
Dr Joan Gomez

Living with Asthma
Dr Robert Youngson

Living with Autism
Fiona Marshall

Living with Crohn's Disease
Dr Joan Gomez

Living with Diabetes
Dr Joan Gomez

Living with Fibromyalgia
Christine Craggs-Hinton

Living with Food Intolerance
Alex Gazzola

Living with Grief
Dr Tony Lake

Living with Heart Disease
Victor Marks, Dr Monica Lewis and
Dr Gerald Lewis

Overcoming Common Problems Series

Overcoming Common Problems

Living with Food Allergy

Alex Gazzola

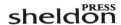

First published in Great Britain in 2006

Sheldon Press
36 Causton Street
London SW1P 4ST

Copyright © Alex Gazzola 2006

The author and publisher have made every effort to ensure that
the external website and email addresses included in this book are
correct and up to date at the time of going to press. The author
and publisher are not responsible for the content, quality or
continuing accessibility of the sites.

All our books are designed to be as helpful and supportive as possible but cannot be used
to diagnose or treat a medical condition, and are not intended to be a substitute for
professional medical advice. If you have or suspect you have a health problem, you
should consult a doctor or other healthcare provider.

British Library Cataloguing-in-Publication Data

A catalogue record for this book is available from the British Library

ISBN-13: 978–0–85969–970–9
ISBN-10: 0–85969–970–6

1 3 5 7 9 10 8 6 4 2

Typeset by Deltatype Limited, Birkenhead, Merseyside
Printed in Great Britain by Ashford Colour Press

Contents

Acknowledgements

Those working in the field of allergy – be it in healthcare, research or support – are, as I learned while researching this book, extremely overstretched. Therefore I'm especially grateful to those who responded to my enquiries and gave generously of what I suspect they had least to give – their time.

Thanks, then, to: Aleks Kinay of the Latex Allergy Support Group; Professor John Warner of the University of Southampton; Carol Rae, Lindsey McManus, Muriel Simmons and all at Allergy UK; allergy dietitian Tanya Wright of Amersham Hospital, Buckinghamshire; Dr Clare Mills of the Institute of Food Research, Norwich; and Dr Taraneh Dean of the David Hide Asthma & Allergy Research Centre, Isle of Wight.

Particular gratitude to Moira Austin, David Reading and all at the Anaphylaxis Campaign.

Thanks due also to: Phillip Hodson, Paul McGee, and Dr Rebecca Knibb of the University of Derby, each of whose ideas and expertise fed Chapter 6; my supportive editor, Fiona Marshall; pharmacist Maeve O'Connell of Boots; Joanne Williams for her observations on Oral Allergy Syndrome (OAS); and all those living with food allergy who have knowingly or otherwise contributed to this book.

Introduction

The food allergy problem

We are guilty of having become somewhat cavalier with the word 'allergy' in the twenty-first century. Many of us now blithely describe ourselves as being 'a bit allergic' to some modern irritant – such as household paint, fragrances or tobacco – while someone of an idle disposition should perhaps not be surprised to hear himself jokingly diagnosed with a 'work allergy'.

But when pressed, most are unsure of what allergy actually is. The often careless media coverage of the subject may be in part responsible, as it might be for the increased numbers self-diagnosing their 'allergies'. Inaccurate diagnoses by alternative therapists, many of whom misuse the word, have compounded the problem. We may not fully understand what it means to be allergic, yet many of us seem to think we are.

Allergies are serious conditions involving unwanted responses of the immune system. Whether sufferers react to pollen, bee stings or latex, for instance, the symptoms – such as rhinitis, nettle rash, eczema – can be debilitating and worrying. At worst, as with asthma, anaphylaxis and anaphylactic shock – or allergic collapse – they have the potential to end life.

This book is concerned with food allergy – an inappropriate, usually rapid and potentially life-threatening response of the body's immune system towards a food component which is harmless to most other people.

Food allergy can cause great misery. But because many mistakenly describe themselves as food-allergic, the seriousness of the condition can be underestimated – with friends and family members, catering workers, even doctors, all sometimes sceptical about genuine cases. If you're food-allergic, the world can seem unsympathetic.

In Britain, this is especially true. Allergy provision on the National Health Service (NHS) is poor. Doctors, who receive little training in food allergies, are struggling with diagnoses. We have only six full-time specialist allergy centres in the country; around 30 allergy consultants. Those fortunate enough to live close to a consultant or clinic usually face nothing more than a waiting list in order to be evaluated. Those outside catchment areas face at best long journeys to appointments, at worst being denied any assessment altogether. Those who can afford it can and do turn to the private sector – where a minefield of practice from excellent to potentially unsafe awaits. And those who can't are often left to manage with minimal support or aftercare.

Estimates vary, but the West is badly affected. In a 2003 Royal College of Physicians report, *Allergy: the Unmet Need*, the range 1.8–3.2 per cent was said to 'underestimate the position' in the UK. Peanut allergy alone affects over 7 per cent of the US population, while the European Federation of Allergy and Airways Diseases Patients' Associations suggests 4 per cent of adults (and 8 per cent of children) in the EU have food allergies. In the last decade, there has been a fivefold increase in adverse reactions to foods.

There's no sign this problem is going away, no reason to suppose the rise will not continue.

How this book will help

Living with Food Allergy aims to inform, support and empower sufferers to cope with everything from the day-to-day practicalities of dealing with their condition to the longer-term implications of allergic illness triggered by food.

Food safety, diet and nutrition are obvious concerns, and these are considered thoroughly. The psychological impact of food allergy is given scant coverage, so Chapter 6 is here to redress the imbalance. Oral Allergy Syndrome, an increasingly common condition usually directly related to hay fever, is another topic about which there is little information, and this is covered in depth too. The comprehensive 'Useful addresses' section will be invaluable to those seeking practical solutions to problems, and includes contact details of all organizations referred to in the text, plus many more.

The avoidance of overly technical information is deliberate. Allergy is a complex branch of medicine, and readers wishing to delve deeper may like to consult some titles in 'Further reading'.

There are three other key points to make:

1 The book is probably best read if the reader has been diagnosed through orthodox means – usually via a doctor and allergy consultant – rather than through a high-street test or alternative therapist. Testing is covered in Appendix 1. However, it is hoped it is of use to anyone who suspects he or she may have a food allergy and to families and friends of those with allergies, as well as to health professionals.

2 The book is written primarily for the adult sufferer, but is also of relevance to older children and young adults – and indeed their parents, families and friends. It is not specifically intended for parents of allergic babies or young children. The diagnosis, management, treatment and prognosis of food allergy in the very young can be specific to that age group, so while some information will help, bear in mind that unless otherwise stated some advice may be unsuited to little ones. Again, other titles can help further.

3 Lastly, the subject of food intolerance – usually characterized by delayed and digestive-based reactions to commonly eaten foods, and often causing chronic and mild, not acute and serious, responses – is not covered here. Adverse reactions to the milk sugar lactose, to food chemicals such as caffeine, to food additives and colourings, and to the wheat protein gluten which triggers coeliac disease, are among those conditions covered by this book's companion title, *Living with Food Intolerance*, by the same publisher and author.

1

What food allergy is

A food allergic reaction is a prompt, inappropriate and adverse response towards an otherwise harmless food component which is triggered by your immune system – the body of cells responsible for defending you from infection.

The substance responsible is called an allergen. Typically, this allergen is a protein – for instance, one of the many proteins found in nuts or fish – which your immune system mistakenly assumes to be a threat. The allergen enters your body through the delicate membranes of the mouth, through the skin, or via ingestion. If you're particularly sensitive, merely the smell of a culprit food can elicit a reaction – the vaporized allergen gaining access through your respiratory system.

Symptoms – which vary according to several factors – include tingling in the mouth, a runny nose, rashes, wheezing and asthma, swelling of the mouth and throat, and vomiting.

Allergic sensitization

For your immune system to deem a protein 'dangerous', it must previously have been exposed to it and subsequently have developed sensitization to it.

Sensitization is essentially an overreaction of your immune system to what it perceives as an 'invader'. Anxious to protect the body, the immune system can respond to a new and suspect protein by manufacturing chemicals called antibodies to tackle it.

The antibodies almost always involved in food allergies are called Immunoglobulin E (IgE). Once formed, IgE antibodies attach themselves to immune cells called mast cells, which tend to be found where your body is most vulnerable to invasion from microbes – such as the nose and lung.

When you subsequently come into contact with an allergen to which you've been sensitized, the allergen and its corresponding IgE antibody bind. This binding causes the host mast cell to be activated

1

and release inflammatory chemicals, such as histamine, in what can be described as an immunological 'call to arms'.

Problems occur when the volume of released chemicals causes unwanted changes in the body. These include the typical symptoms of food allergy – swelling, rashes, diarrhoea and vomiting – all aimed at flushing out the 'invader'. Unfortunately for you, these reactions can be uncomfortable, distressing and at worst life-threatening.

Age and sensitization

Allergic sensitization often happens when people are very young, before the immune system is mature enough to deal with the complex proteins typically associated with food allergy. A child can be fed an allergen directly, consume it in the mother's breast milk, or even receive it before birth through the placental bloodstream. There is evidence that creams used in infancy containing food proteins – such as nappy creams – can sensitize children to the source food.

However, sensitization or the emergence of food allergy symptoms in young adulthood and in later life is becoming more common, for reasons which are unclear. Sometimes, in food-industry workers, occupational exposure is to blame – for instance, those employed in flour factories and exposed to inhaled allergens may become sensitized and later react to wheat.

The allergic march

Following sensitization, the progression of allergic illness through life is difficult to predict.

Childhood food allergies can disappear permanently, diminish in severity, remain unchanged, or diminish or disappear then re-emerge in adulthood, sometimes in a new form. Most young children outgrow sensitivities to milk, eggs, wheat and soya, for instance, but only about one in five will do likewise to nuts. Fish allergy also tends to be retained into adulthood.

Later-onset food allergies are more likely to be permanent afflictions which tend not to worsen, and in some cases may improve.

Causes

Although we understand *how* people become sensitized and allergic to food, the reasons *why* remain unclear.

What we do know is that some are more susceptible than others to food allergy, and that this is due to atopy – the hereditary and genetic predisposition to suffer from any allergic illness.

If you suffer from allergies other than food allergies, or if your parents suffered from any allergic conditions, it is more likely that you will develop food allergies. That said, most individuals with allergic tendencies do not develop food allergies, and some non-atopic people and those from non-atopic families do (especially in infancy).

Other factors

There are undoubtedly considerations other than genetic to take into account, given that studies on identical twins show they often present dissimilar allergic status. Several ideas have been suggested, and a combination may be at work.

The hygiene hypothesis

This holds that, because of our modern aversion to dirt and tendency to disinfect our homes excessively, we are no longer exposing ourselves to the 'stimulus' of the largely benevolent everyday bacteria which are thought to prime the immune system's protective mechanisms. In the absence of such helpful triggers, the immune system instead turns its attention towards other 'intruders' – food proteins. Those brought up in natural, rural environments, exposed daily to unsanitized farm life, show lower incidences of allergy than people reared in clean, centrally heated urban homes.

Smaller families

With couples now tending to have only one or two children in Western societies, we're less likely to be exposed to infections 'brought home' by older siblings as would have occurred in previous generations with larger families. Reduced sharing of childhood infections could again be resulting in an under-exercised – and therefore malfunctioning – immune system.

Altered gut flora

According to research, allergic children have lower levels of beneficial probiotic bacteria in their intestines. It's uncertain whether this may be a likely cause or consequence of allergy, but it has been suggested the overuse of broad-spectrum antibiotics has unbalanced our internal ecosystems, possibly compromising immunity.

Altered nutrition

A low intake of fruit and vegetables is now typical of the Western diet, leaving us deficient in nutrients. The consequential increase in protein consumption (and therefore more potential food triggers) could also be a factor.

Further, foods previously unknown to us are now nothing more than an air flight away, with an array of exotica available at most supermarkets – each with its own collection of potential allergens with which we may be ill-equipped to cope.

Traces in our foods of pesticides, fertilizers and growth hormones used in modern farming practice may also be clouding the picture.

Pollutants and chemicals

Environmental pollution, household chemicals and toiletries, and exposure to tobacco smoke could, theoretically, be suppressing correct immunological responses in some.

Pollution could also be problematic for plants. The increase in allergy to fruits and vegetables may be due to plants producing greater amounts of allergenic proteins as a defence against greater environmental stresses.

The prime allergens

According to the 2000 report *Adverse Reactions to Food and Food Ingredients*, published by the Committee on Toxicity of Chemicals in Food, Consumer Products and the Environment, 90 per cent of food-allergic reactions in Western European children are caused by milk, eggs, wheat, soya, peanuts and tree nuts.

The same report states that around 90 per cent of food-allergic reactions in adults are caused by peanuts, tree nuts, fish and shellfish. However, this figure is now likely to be an overestimate, given the increase in Oral Allergy Syndrome – a relatively new condition among young adults characterized by usually mild allergies to fruits, vegetables, spices, seeds, nuts and herbs.

4

Among the most dangerous food allergens – often dubbed the 'big eight', as they're the most common – are these:

- peanuts;
- tree nuts (such as Brazils, cashews, walnuts);
- fish;
- shellfish;
- milk and dairy foods;
- eggs (yolk and white);
- wheat;
- soya.

The following, while generally rarer, are potentially equally serious:

- legumes, such as chickpeas, peas, lentils, and especially lupin;
- seeds, such as sesame, sunflower and poppy;
- mustard;
- celery (and celeriac);
- kiwis, apples, and the rose stone fruits (peaches, cherries, plums).

However, it is perfectly possible to be mildly allergic to peanut and apple, for instance, and dangerously allergic to an infrequently troublesome food, such as sweet potato. There are almost 200 foods on record which have caused reactions, and of varying degrees of severity. Sadly, food allergy remains a relatively imprecise science.

There is no easy answer, too, to the question of the quantity of food required to produce a reaction. Around 50mg of egg is often needed in an egg-sensitive adult. However, as little as 0.1mg of peanut can incite a response in the peanut allergic.

Ditto the issue of cooked versus uncooked food. Roasting nuts, for instance, appears to increase their allergenic potential, and in the case of pecan nuts can even create new allergens. Meanwhile, some egg-allergics can tolerate processed eggs, and possibly hard-boiled eggs, but not lightly cooked eggs. Some react to raw fish, some to cooked, and some to both. Cooking or otherwise processing fruits and vegetables tends to make them less threatening – although many who react to celery do so to both cooked and raw forms.

Non-allergens

Although allergic reactions to most foods are possible, certain food components, many essential to our diet, do not cause them.

You cannot be allergic to the vitamin C or salt in a food, for instance, or any other vitamin or essential mineral. Ditto to water, to fats or oils, to alcohol, or to simple sugars, such as table sugar, glucose or lactose (milk sugar).

It is proteins which cause the vast majority of food allergies. Reactions to non-protein components are likely to be food intolerances or other sensitivities.

A worldwide disease

Food allergy is largely a problem of the developed nations – North America, Europe, Australasia and Japan. There is variation in the culprits among individual nationals; the 'big eight', however, tend to be pronounced in most countries where food allergy is endemic. The more popular a food is, the more likely an allergy to that food will become apparent.

For instance, Americans, great consumers of peanut butter, are plagued with severe peanut allergies, as well as a corn allergy problem.

The Japanese are likelier than others to suffer from allergies to rice and to buckwheat (used in their popular 'soba' noodles).

Scandinavians, who have a diet rich in seafood, endure high levels of cod allergy, while Mediterraneans tend to be more vulnerable to allergies to lentils and pulses than other nationals. Central Europeans such as the Swiss and Germans are at increased risk of celery allergy. Lupin allergy is an emerging problem for the French, who use it widely as a flour.

2

Symptoms and reactions

Food-allergic symptoms and reactions are many and varied, and can be localized or systemic.

Localized reactions are confined to the point of contact with the allergen; with food, this is usually the lips, mouth and throat.

Systemic reactions affect all parts of the body, and are usually more dangerous.

Symptoms tend to be acute – that is, they come on rapidly, are pronounced and short-lived. Chronic allergic illness – which is of gradual onset, is of slow progression, and is long-lasting – is only rarely triggered by food allergy, but more commonly can be exacerbated by it.

Reactions of the skin

Urticaria is the most common acute food-allergic reaction of the skin – although it can have other causes, such as sun exposure. It is a rash characterized by raised swellings called weals, maddening itchiness (or pruritus), and reddening or flushing (erythema), occurring within minutes of exposure to the culprit food. Also called hives or nettle-rash, urticaria is brought on by histamine release into the skin's layers, causing microscopic blood vessels to seep fluid into the skin's tissues. Food allergy is unlikely to be involved in chronic urticaria.

Around half of acute urticarial food reactions are accompanied by *angioedema* – localized swelling or puffiness – which occurs when blood vessel leakage is more severe. Acute angioedema in the absence of urticaria is possible, but uncommon. Chronic angioedema – a serious symptom – is unlikely to be food-allergic in origin.

Atopic dermatitis or *eczema* is a collection of chronic inflammatory and itchy, and sometimes flaky, weepy and scaly skin conditions, particularly prevalent in the young, and often associated with other allergic disorders, such as asthma. Food allergy may be involved and can exacerbate eczema, but other factors – such as toiletries, temperature extremes, and food intolerances to wheat, milk and eggs – are likelier. Worsening of eczema symptoms in the

7

days following an urticarial or angioedemal food-allergic episode is often reported.

Reactions of the respiratory system

Inflammation of the mucous membranes of the nose, called *rhinitis*, is a common, minor food-allergic response, while a runny nose, called *rhinorrhoea*, is a symptom of increased nasal secretion. Both are more likely when culprit foods are inhaled or sniffed rather than consumed. Bloodshot, watery eyes (allergic conjunctivitis) and sneezing may also occur.

Chronic rhinitis – or perennial allergic rhinitis – is associated with pollens, dust mites, moulds or pets.

Wheezing and shortness of breath are symptoms of *asthma*, a narrowing of the bronchial airways in the lung caused by inflammation, which can occur in more serious food-allergic responses, especially in chronic asthma or otherwise atopic patients. Wheezing may be caused or exacerbated by angioedema in the throat. Chronic asthma may be caused or exacerbated by food allergy, but other causative factors are likelier.

Reactions of the gastrointestinal system

Nausea, abdominal pain and vomiting can be symptoms when the food culprits cause internal irritation and inflammation of the gullet (oesophagus) and stomach. Although there are other causes of such symptoms – bacteria, poisons – vomiting in combination with skin or respiratory symptoms implies a severe allergic reaction.

Oral Allergy Syndrome (OAS)

This is an allergy to fruits, vegetables, herbs, spices, seeds and nuts which is restricted to the oral cavity – the lips, the mouth, the tongue and sometimes the throat.

Itching, urticaria and angioedema are the prime symptoms of OAS if the food is eaten, usually within minutes of consumption. However, merely preparing raw produce can trigger mild respiratory or conjunctival symptoms if you're exposed to traces of vaporized juices, and peeling fruit and vegetables can bring on urticaria on the hands too. Wheezing is possible if the angioedema spreads to the throat, but the symptoms are not normally life-threatening – in fact, they can be so mild that sufferers may ignore or barely be conscious of them.

Pollen–food cross-reactions

OAS is usually a consequence of hay fever – an allergy to one or more spores or pollens, such as birch or grass pollens – the symptoms of which include sneezing, runny eyes and nose, itchy nose and occasionally light wheezing, headache and tiredness.

If you're sensitized to the proteins in pollens, food reactions might later develop because similar proteins happen to be also present in many plant foods. Your immune system, 'assuming' that you have bitten into a mouthful of allergenic pollen, reacts accordingly.

These responses – where previous sensitization to one allergen or food effectively results in sensitization and symptoms emerging to others – are known as *cross-reactions*. With pollen–food cross-reactions, many fruits and vegetables can be involved (see box p. 10).

There appears to be a proportional link between the ripeness of a fruit and the severity of the response. Peeling a fruit may sometimes reduce the reaction. Because the proteins involved in pollen–food cross-reactions tend to be fragile, cooking or otherwise processing the host food can destroy them, rendering the food tolerable. There are possible exceptions, though – such as nuts, celery and some spices – and the subject is further explored in Chapter 4, part II.

Since the culprit proteins are usually deactivated on contact with the stomach's digestive juices, gastrointestinal reactions are unlikely.

Incidence and prevalence

Hay fever is seasonal and you will only endure symptoms when relevant plants or trees are pollinating. However, once you are sensitized to pollens, any associated food-allergic cross-reactions will occur all year round – although out of season they are usually milder, and in season stronger, especially during high pollen counts.

Pollen-related OAS is rare in children, but more frequently seen in older teenagers and young adults, in which group it is the commonest food-allergic manifestation. Often, there is improvement in middle age and beyond.

In the UK, around 15 per cent of the population is pollen sensitive. Of that figure, around 90 per cent react to grass and 25 per cent to birch – the two most important allergenic pollen types in this country. Up to 90 per cent of birch-pollen sensitives react to raw fruits and vegetables, such as apple, carrot and celery.

Pollen–food cross-reactions

Some reactions are still being recorded, so this list cannot be exhaustive. Individuals with OAS often stumble across new problem foods. Any you react to indicate you're more likely to also react to close family members – see Appendix 2.

- *Birch (also alder, elm and hazel), Northern Europe, America and Asia, season: spring.* Most birch-pollen sensitives have oral allergies, potentially to many foods, including avocado, the carrot family (carrots, celery, parsley), the nightshade family (pepper, potato, tomato), pineapple, kiwi, the rose family (apple, pear, peach, plum), spinach, and many nuts and spices.
- *Grass, worldwide, season: summer.* Few grass-pollen sensitives have OAS, but reported reactions include apple, kiwi, melon, orange, peanut and other legumes, Swiss chard, tomato and grass grains (wheat, rye).
- *Mugwort or ragwort, Northern and Central Europe, season: summer/autumn.* Reactions to apple, the carrot family (especially celery), the daisy family (camomile, sunflower seeds) and the melon family (courgette, cucumber) are possible, as are those to spices (pepper, poppy seed).
- *Ragweed, North America, season: late summer/autumn.* The daisy and melon families, and possibly banana.

More predictable cross-reactions, such as those between pine pollen and pine nuts, are also recognized. There may be a link between rape seed pollen and other members of the mustard family, specifically mustard itself. Honeys containing pollens can cause symptoms too, but these are rare and usually mild.

Elsewhere the picture varies, mainly depending on local flora. In Germany and Scandinavia, for instance, birch-pollen allergy is more widespread, but it is less so in southern Europe, which has few birch woods. In Italy, for example, hay fever is largely caused by grass pollen, and oral allergies to tomatoes and melons are more common.

Unfortunately, it is possible to become sensitized to a non-native pollen during a foreign trip in peak season. For instance, an atopic individual visiting North America can become sensitized to ragweed. Returning home, he or she will not experience hay fever symptoms (there is no ragweed in the UK) but may suffer ragweed–food cross-reactions.

Note that although pollen–food reactions tend not to be serious, if you suffer from an allergy to a fruit, vegetable or nut in the absence of any pollen sensitivity, the reactions are more likely to be severe. For instance, apple or peach allergies related to hay fever are less of a threat than apple or peach allergies unrelated to hay fever. Serious fruit allergies are less common in northern Europe, and more so in southern nations such as Italy and Spain.

Other cross-reactions

Pollen aside, there are other sensitizers which can cross-react with foods.

Mould spores

Those sensitized to mould or fungal spores – both external and internal – sometimes report mild oral reactions to mushrooms, yeast-based spreads, mycoprotein/Quorn, and brewed, fermented or matured foods such as mouldy cheeses or vinegars.

Bird feathers

A cross-reaction in those allergic to bird feathers is possible with egg yolk.

Dust mites

The droppings of the house dust mite are highly allergenic, and many people respond to them – asthma, eczema and especially rhinitis are common symptoms. In rare cases, sufferers can react, sometimes severely, to kiwi, papaya, shellfish and possibly soya, due to coincidental similarities of certain allergens.

Latex

Allergy to latex (natural rubber) is common among healthcare workers regularly exposed to latex gloves; around 7 per cent suffer. The condition is rarer in the wider population (under 1 per cent); but those undergoing repeated surgical interventions are more at risk. Around half of sufferers experience cross-reactions with foods, which tend to be tropical fruits. Avocado appears to be the commonest culprit, followed by banana, chestnut and kiwi, but reactions to buckwheat, cherry, fig, mango, melon, papaya, passion fruit, peach, potato, tomato, and nuts and legumes are reported too, and this list is growing. Reactions to latex – and its cross-reacting foods – can be systemic and serious.

Food–food cross-reactions

So far we have looked at allergic conditions where non-foods have been the primary sensitizers, but of course foods themselves regularly sensitize individuals, as is usually the case with the 'big eight'– peanuts, tree nuts, fish, shellfish, dairy, eggs, wheat and soya.

Allergies to one or more of these mean you're more likely to experience reactions to foods related to them. In the case of the legumes soya and peanut, for instance, you may be more susceptible to other legumes such as lupin and chickpeas. An allergy to wheat leaves you more at risk of allergies to grains closely related to it, including rye and barley.

Tree nuts and peanuts are unusual in that they're the best example of foods which tend to cross-react with some outsiders as well as 'siblings'. Most tree nuts are not closely related, and yet becoming sensitized to one can make you vulnerable to reactions to others, and to peanut, which botanically speaking is a legume, not a nut. Equally, in reverse, sensitization to the peanut leaves you not only more likely to react to other legumes, but to tree nuts too.

It's difficult to put a figure on the risks for individual nuts, because there are many allergens to consider. However, as a random example, one study of 1,000 peanut- and tree nut-allergic patients showed that 45 per cent could tolerate almond.

Other, albeit much rarer, cross-reactions between unrelated foods are still being explored. Some of these 'clusters of hypersensitivity' are notable for their cross-familial diversity, such as the grouping consisting of hazelnuts, kiwi fruit, poppy seeds, rye and sesame. The Institute of Food Research's Allergen Database, at foodallergens. ifr.ac.uk, has many other curious examples, mostly related to pollen sensitivities.

With most animal-sourced foods, cross-reactions are common. Sensitization to hen's eggs is virtually tantamount to sensitization to all eggs, as the culprit proteins are common to all. If you're allergic to cow's milk, there's a greater than 90 per cent likelihood you'll react to goat's, but slightly less to sheep's milk.

Similarly, if you've been sensitized to one fish, you're likely to experience reactions with others; and it's a similar situation with crustaceans (crab, lobster, prawn) and molluscs (clam, cockle, scallop).

Appendix 2 lists plant and seafood families.

Anaphylaxis

Of all the allergic reactions, anaphylaxis is the most extreme.

Food-allergic reactions considered at the beginning of the chapter – of the skin, and respiratory and gastrointestinal systems – can be and normally are all involved, but anaphylactic reactions progress further. Typical symptoms of food-induced anaphylaxis, approximately in the order they usually present themselves, include some but not necessarily all of the following:

- flushing, itching and urticaria, especially around the face and mouth initially – but then often progressing elsewhere on the body;
- swelling (oedema), especially around the face, oral cavity and throat – but potentially more widespread;
- a blocked nose and sneezing;
- hoarseness and difficulty speaking;
- wheeziness and laboured breathing (more pronounced in asthmatics);
- difficulty swallowing;

- an increased pulse or palpitations (tachycardia);
- gastric pain, nausea, vomiting;
- a sense of impending doom; anxiety, panic, confusion, disorientation;
- lower abdominal pain, diarrhoea, incontinence;
- weakness, dizziness and 'floppiness', caused by a sudden drop in blood pressure;
- circulatory collapse and unconsciousness – anaphylactic shock.

Anaphylactic reactions usually come on rapidly – within minutes or even seconds of exposure – or rarely quite slowly, up to an hour or more later. Also, the progression from mild oral symptoms to dangerous respiratory and cardiovascular breakdown can be extremely quick, or less typically much slower.

Older children and adults are more likely to suffer from anaphylaxis – it rarely affects babies and young children. Even a trace quantity of almost any food can cause it; the main culprits are listed on p. 5, but peanuts and tree nuts are undoubtedly the prime danger foods.

It is rare that OAS progresses to anaphylaxis – only 2 per cent of OAS sufferers have reported an episode, and these have typically involved nuts, celery, kiwi or the rose family fruits.

Latex allergy can cause anaphylaxis, and other non-food triggers include insect stings and snake bites.

Reactions to drugs like penicillin are possible too.

Risk factors

Anaphylaxis can kill – through asphyxiation because of swelling of the throat, cardiac arrest and circulatory collapse, or a fatal asthma attack. So how do you know whether you're at risk?

Some doctors consider anyone allergic to tree nuts, peanuts, seeds and seafood – no matter how mild their symptoms – to be at potential risk.

If you've had severe allergic responses in the past, this can also increase your chances of suffering an anaphylactic reaction. The same applies if you're asthmatic – in which case your reaction is more likely to be life-threatening.

Having exercised prior to exposure can also 'tip over' a moderate reaction into an anaphylactic one. Sometimes, exercise following a particular food – even as long as a day later – can be directly responsible for triggering a reaction. This rare condition is called exercise-induced anaphylaxis – and the cause can be difficult to pinpoint because no reaction is experienced from exposure to the allergen in the absence of exercise. Prawns, celery and wheat (gluten) are some of the foods implicated in exercise-induced anaphylaxis; the condition appears to be commonest in young female athletes.

Exposure to heat (a sauna, for instance) or even cold can worsen a reaction. In some, having taken aspirins or other drugs can have an exacerbating effect too. A high dose of the culprit allergen – perhaps when 'disguised' in an unfamiliar food – can push a reaction over the edge, and if alcohol is involved, the reaction will be speedier, and your response times and judgement may be impaired.

Unfortunately there have been a number of cases where anaphylactic reactions have occurred out of the blue, with no previous warning. Sadly, susceptibility to anaphylaxis is normally lifelong.

Anaphylactic reactions, like all others, respond to prompt and appropriate treatment.

Allergy-like reactions

Some strong reactions to food may not be allergic. Most are covered in greater depth in this book's companion title, *Living with Food Intolerance* (Sheldon, 2005).

Food-induced rhinitis/conjunctivitis

Runny nose/eyes triggered by certain strong foods – horseradish, raw garlic, spices, chillies, for instance. Food rich in histamine – such as fermented or matured foods (sauerkraut, cheeses, wines) – can effect similar reactions.

False food allergy

IgE antibodies are not involved here; instead the mast cells are activated directly, releasing histamine, causing a reaction which appears allergic. It is rare, and rarely fatal. Shellfish, strawberries, tomatoes, chocolate, citrus fruit, egg, pork, some

---

food additives (colourings, preservatives) and aspirin are typical culprits.

Sulphite-induced asthma

About 1–2 per cent of asthmatics react to sulphite preservatives (E221–8) in foods such as cold meats and fish, alcoholic beverages, dried fruits and prepared salads, sometimes severely enough to trigger anaphylaxis. The cause is sulphur dioxide (E220), which is released from the sulphites when they're consumed. The mechanism is not understood.

Food toxicity

Wild fish and shellfish can absorb toxic algae, resulting in unpleasant gastrointestinal and feverish symptoms should you then eat the contaminated food – something often mistaken for fish allergy.

Scombroid poisoning

If oily fish, such as tuna and mackerel, is improperly stored, its natural histamine levels can increase alarmingly. Cooking will not destroy the histamine, which imparts a metallic or peppery taste. Symptoms include urticaria, oedema, headaches and diarrhoea.

3

Reaction management

Obviously it is better to steer clear of your known triggers and possibly other potentially troublesome foods, and the next two chapters will look closely at avoidance tactics. Nevertheless, dealing with reactions is an inescapable fact of life, no matter how vigilant you happen to be, so it is vital you learn how best to deal with them when they occur.

Although there is no cure for food allergy, there are medicines to help you manage reactions – *when they happen accidentally*. Never take these pre-emptively before consuming a food to which you normally react in the hope of preventing a reaction – this is dangerous. Always play safe.

Antihistamines

Antihistamines counteract the effects of histamine – one of the principal chemicals released in an allergic reaction.

Although antihistamines are known more for controlling allergic conditions such as hay fever, they can be effective in tackling the symptoms of mild food allergies. Many are available over the counter and your doctor or pharmacist can advise on which may suit you.

Loratadine (found in Clarityn) and cetirizine (Benadryl, Piriteze and Zirtek) are two which may be recommended. Both are non-sedating, meaning they're unlikely to make you feel drowsy. Chlorpheniramine (Piriton) is an 'old school' antihistamine, which can make you sleepy. There are occasional advantages to sleep-inducing antihistamines – for instance, if you suffer a mild reaction late in the evening which is likely to agitate you at a time when you're hoping to wind down.

Most come in tablet or liquid form. Tablets are easy to carry, but syrups can be taken without water. Syrups, usually sweetened, tend to be favoured by children, to whom a precise dose can be given. Some 'fast-melt' antihistamines are now available, which simply dissolve in the mouth. In terms of performance, there is little to

17

choose between them.

Liquid antihistamines may be prescribed should you be at risk of anaphylaxis, but they are not enough to manage a systemic reaction, and in this case adrenaline is usually needed too (see p. 19).

Contraindications

Antihistamines may not suit everybody. For instance, if you have diabetes or a sugar intolerance, syrups may be inadvisable. Some antihistamines should not be taken by young children, or those with decreased liver or kidney function. Pregnant or nursing women are often advised to avoid certain kinds; the safer ones tend to be the older varieties, but always speak to your doctor for guidance.

Let your pharmacist know if you are taking other medicines or have chronic or short-term conditions. Groups who should be vigilant include the elderly, those living with epilepsy, glaucoma or asthma, and those with cardiovascular disease or high blood pressure.

Some side effects are possible, including dry mouth, restlessness or headaches. Always read labels carefully.

Inhalers

If you're asthmatic, you'll already have drugs to manage your condition. Asthma drugs are either preventers or relievers. Preventers counteract the inflammation in the lungs which triggers the contraction of the muscles surrounding the airways that causes asthmatic symptoms. Relievers relax those muscles, thereby opening up the airways, easing discomfort and breathing.

Preventers should be taken as prescribed by your healthcare provider, but serve no direct purpose in treating acute food-allergic reactions – although the better your asthma is managed through preventative medication, the less severe any reactions are likely to be. If you feel your management of asthma is poor and could be improved upon, make an appointment with your doctor or consultant.

Relievers, though, in the form of inhalers (or bronchodilators) can help, and can be used in conjunction with antihistamines in the management of all allergic reactions to food, including those typically involved in OAS.

Remember that symptoms of wheezing can signify a more serious reaction that may require adrenaline treatment, and that as an asthmatic you are more at risk.

Managing mild or OAS-related reactions

Experiencing the characteristic oral tingling of a mild food allergic reaction? Here's what to do:

- spit out any food at once, into your hand or preferably a napkin;
- rinse your mouth (and then eyes if necessary) thoroughly with plain water, taking someone with you if you use public facilities;
- take any medication such as antihistamines or inhalers, and keep them near;
- if you're alone, stay close to a phone;
- rest, stay calm, and let the reaction pass, as it should within 30 minutes to an hour;
- do not panic or try to make yourself sick;
- keep your body cool, not warm, and relieve any mild heat rash by fanning air onto affected areas – avoid scratching;
- use an eyewash such as Optrex if your eyes are irritated;
- avoid alcohol, taking exercise or hot baths in the hours after a reaction;
- later, review your management of the reaction – is there anything you could have done better?

Remember that OAS reactions are rarely dangerous, but if your reactions have been getting steadily worse, speak to your doctor or allergist.

Adrenaline auto-injector pens

These are one-use automated drug delivery systems each containing a dose of adrenaline and a concealed, spring-loaded needle. They can only be prescribed by your doctor or an allergy consultant, should either consider you at risk of anaphylaxis, for which emergency they are the front-line treatment.

During an allergic reaction, the body's adrenal glands produce increased volumes of the hormone adrenaline (epinephrine). Adrenaline constricts your blood vessels, preventing them from leaking and increasing your blood pressure; it also stimulates your heart, relaxes the pulmonary muscles to improve your breathing, and helps reduce facial swelling.

However, during an extreme reaction the body can be so overwhelmed that its ability to produce sufficient adrenaline is curbed, which is why an adrenaline injection – delivered into the thigh muscle – can help stabilize life-threatening symptoms until emergency services arrive.

Which pen?

There are two: the more established EpiPen, distributed by ALK-Abelló (www.epipen.co.uk), and the newer Anapen, from Lincoln Medical (www.anapen.co.uk).

Both come in two strengths. The adult pens deliver a 0.3mg dose of adrenaline, the children's 0.15mg – although children weighing over 30kg will be prescribed adult pens.

The principal difference between the two is in their mode of use: the EpiPen requires a 'jabbing' motion to trigger its spring-loaded mechanism, while the Anapen features a firing button. The EpiPen's needle is also slightly longer than the Anapen's, so the latter may be less suited to bulkier individuals.

You should carry two pens if you're at risk of a severe reaction.

When to use one?

If you've experienced severe reactions previously, know you've been exposed to your trigger, and symptoms have begun, most doctors would recommend that you use your adrenaline at once, even while your symptoms may still be mild.

If you have no experience of an anaphylactic reaction but have been prescribed an injector pen as a precautionary measure, then distinguishing a mild food reaction and the onset of a serious reaction can be difficult – often, the initial symptoms are the same. Ask yourself these questions:

- do symptoms seem more severe than ever before – and are they steadily worsening?

- are there signs of all-over symptoms – such as rashes or itchiness around the body?
- is your throat tightening and your voice hoarse, or are you coughing or choking?
- are you wheezing or experiencing asthma symptoms?
- are you experiencing difficulty breathing or swallowing?
- are you feeling sick, dizzy, weak or faint?
- do you have severe abdominal pain?

Each can signify the onset of an anaphylactic response, in which case you should use your adrenaline pen immediately.

If experience tells you your symptoms seem mild and stable, take action appropriate to an OAS reaction or as directed by your medical advisor, but stay alert to any worsening of your symptoms and primed to act accordingly.

If you're unsure, the consensus opinion is to use your adrenaline. The drug is safe, the needle virtually painless, and you should not experience any long-lasting side effects if you use it when not strictly necessary. The worse seem to be short term – a 'rush of blood to the head', a heightened feeling of stress or anxiety, sweating or shaking, and a stronger heartbeat.

If you think you may have been exposed to your allergen, but do not have symptoms yet, take some antihistamines and remain calm and alert. It is better not to inject unless and until symptoms begin; after all, it is possible you were not exposed to the allergen, or even sufficient quantities of it, or – much less likely – that you have outgrown the allergy.

How to use one?

As soon as you realize you're having what appears to be the making of a serious allergic response, act immediately – never deny the problem, or question whether you're overreacting.

If you are with other people, the first steps of the emergency procedure are to tell them what is happening, take out your injector pen, and ask someone to call 999 and report that you are having a suspected anaphylactic reaction.

If you're feeling faint, it's usually better to lie on your back and elevate your legs – prop them on a chair or against a wall, or get someone to hold them up – in order to help get blood to your heart and head and raise your blood pressure. If you're feeling faint and nauseous, it's safer to lie on your side to eliminate the risk of choking on vomit.

If you have acute asthmatic symptoms, however, it's sometimes better to sit upright with your arms anchored so that your neck and shoulder muscles can be used for breathing. That said, it is far more important to sustain blood pressure than it is to deal with wheezing. Anaphylactic death from low blood pressure can be quick.

Then, when using an EpiPen, hold the pen in your dominant fist like a dagger. With your free hand, remove the grey safety cap and jab the black tip firmly into your upper outer thigh. You'll hear a click which tells you the needle has been deployed.

When using an Anapen, remove the black needle cap and the firing button safety cap, hold the Anapen against your outer thigh, and press the red button to deploy the needle.

The rest of the procedure is identical for both pens. Hold the pen in position for ten seconds to allow the full dose to be dispensed. Then withdraw the pen (some fluid will remain), set it aside, and massage the injected area for a further ten seconds. You should feel the benefits almost at once.

If you are alone, inject first and then call emergency services. If you can, then call a friend or family member to join you. Note the time – when they arrive, medical staff will need to know when you injected. Don't at any stage leap up off the floor if you've been lying down; only get up very slowly and carefully, and lie back down if you still feel dizzy.

Note that auto-injectors should be used only on the upper outer portion of the thigh – anywhere else on the body can be dangerous – and that you can if necessary inject through clothing, including denim, but you may have difficulty with leather.

The Anaphylaxis Campaign has a video featuring a demonstration in the use of adrenaline injector pens. The websites of the two manufacturers carry instructions; ALK-Abelló's has a video clip.

After you use one

Remain calm. Take a dose of antihistamines if you can and haven't already, and use your asthma reliever if you need to. There are no additional risks involved in using all three forms of medication in combination. Because the body rapidly eliminates adrenaline, you may need a second injection ten minutes after the first if symptoms don't improve or help is slow in arriving.

If it does not interfere with self-treatment, which should be your priority, save a portion of the food which you feel triggered your response – or better still, ask someone to put it aside or store it in a freezer if it's degradable, as you may need it later to identify the culprit.

When paramedics arrive, hand used pens to them. They will assess you, possibly give you more treatment and in all likelihood take you to Accident and Emergency (A&E).

At A&E, you'll be treated further, possibly with antihistamines, corticosteroids (which fight inflammation), adrenaline (via injection or a nebulizer) and in extreme cases oxygen and intravenous fluids. Ideally, you'll be monitored for up to six hours – but at least four. This is important, because repeat or 'rebound' reactions – called biphasic reactions – can occur hours (even days) after initial exposure. This occurs when you have swallowed significant quantities of allergens which are resistant to breakdown in the body, such as peanut allergens, as they may continue to be absorbed through the digestive system for some time.

If you are discharged very early, ask to stay. If that's impossible due to bed or staff shortages, it's a good idea to remain on site in a waiting area for several hours. Be aware of the possibility of a secondary reaction, and remember to obtain replacement injectors before you leave. You may also be given additional medication which you should take as directed.

After the reaction

Don't exert yourself. For several days avoid alcohol and temperature extremes (such as hot baths) and take as much rest as possible.

Once you're recovered, review what happened and your emergency response procedure. What didn't go smoothly? What can you improve? Is there anything you can learn in order to help you next time? Use the support groups if you need to or speak to your consultant.

If the cause of the reaction remains a puzzle, it's important to find out how it occurred. This can be a laborious task, but it's vital you pursue it until you get a definitive answer.

If you suspect that a contaminant in a food product you thought was safe may have triggered your reaction, or that a manufacturer has made a packaging or labelling error, report it to the manufacturer and/or the store from which the product was bought. They will want to know packaging information, such as batch number, product code, place of purchase and expiry dates, so hold on to this. Manufacturers are normally co-operative, but the allergy charities can advise if you encounter recalcitrance. If contamination is suspected, the food should be lab-tested, and a positive outcome should then be reported to the charities so they can send warnings to their members.

In the event of a negative outcome to your particular allergen, you need to consider other possibilities – including having developed an allergy to a new food. Appendix 2 on food families might suggest a possible cross-reaction, or else speak to your doctor or allergist who may be able to deduce the culprit or suggest further tests to identify it.

If you were dining at a restaurant, make an appointment to speak with the chef in order to carefully go through the ingredients of your meal, if only to eliminate the possibility of your having a previously unknown allergy. If you received guarantees that your meal would be free of your allergen, and lab-testing on a saved sample disproves this, you may have grounds to take action.

The allergy charities can advise on legal matters should you have been harmed by a reaction that was not your fault, and the Anaphylaxis Campaign will suggest laboratories which undertake food testing. However, it's a good idea in the first instance to get in touch with the environmental health department at your local authority, whose food enforcement officer should be able to advise and if necessary take up your case.

Injector pen management and care

Your EpiPen or Anapen is a life-saving medicine which you should treat with great care.

First, and most essentially, always carry it with you. Very few deaths annually are due to food-mediated anaphylaxis – around ten – but most of these occur when adrenaline is not available for administration in the early stages of a reaction. Carry it in the *same* place always, so you, and others, know where to find it. Several manufacturers produce protective carrying cases for your pens – see 'Useful addresses'.

Read the instructions that come with your pen, and reread them frequently to consolidate your understanding. Ask a nurse at your local surgery to give you a refresher lesson from time to time.

Check your adrenaline and its expiry date regularly. Adrenaline which is more than three months past its expiry date will be ineffective. Healthy adrenaline should be clear and colourless. If it's cloudy or yellow it should not be used. EpiPen users can register with ALK-Abelló's expiry-date alert service to receive timely letter or e-mail reminders to have injectors replaced.

Adrenaline can degrade in hot or cold conditions, so protect it from direct sunlight or hot cars, and never store in the refrigerator.

Friends and family

Everyone close to you needs to be made aware of your condition and the ways you manage it.

Don't overwhelm people at first. Think back to how it took you a while to get used to your diagnosis and medication and their implications – it's the same for your loved ones. 'Train' them gradually. For example, first make them aware of what your food allergy is, where your culprit may be hidden, and how even a trace amount can affect you. Show them your medical bracelet, if you wear one.

You also need to tell them of the signs and symptoms of anaphylaxis: refer them to relevant sections of this book.

Then, show them your medication. When you think they're ready, introduce them to your emergency procedure and your injector pens. It's important you do this, as knowing there are people looking out for you who can assist in an emergency is reassuring; most will be only too glad to help relieve you of some of the stress.

Injector pen suppliers offer 'trainer' pens which are useful in demonstrating to friends and relatives how your pens work – these can also be useful to practise with. Distinguishing colour aside, trainer pens are identical to the real thing, but lack adrenaline or a needle. ALK-Abelló offers a lifeline patient training pack which includes a trainer with patient information and a poster for your office or school.

Action plans

If you suffer such a serious reaction that you're unable to administer your own medication, others need to step in.

As well as educating them – through this book, other materials, and your own instruction – it helps to give them an action plan of what to do in an emergency. Because each individual is different, an all-suitable template is not appropriate: you should formulate a plan specific to you with the assistance of your doctor or allergy specialist.

An action plan could include:

- details of your allergy, your typical symptoms on exposure, and signs of an anaphylactic response;
- how you should be positioned or assisted during a reaction;
- how to check your airways, and how you can be helped with your breathing it it's laboured (the handle of a spoon slid carefully over the length of the tongue and then lightly depressed and held in place can ease breathing, for instance);
- where your medication, including your adrenaline, is kept, and how it should be used if you're unconscious;
- an instruction to call 999, and what the emergency services should be told: for instance, that a patient is suffering a suspected anaphylactic reaction; that adrenaline has been/is being administered; the address and postcode of the patient's location (include on the sheet those of your home, study or workplace and anywhere else you commonly frequent);
- follow-up instructions: that someone should wait outside to direct emergency services; that a second injection can be administered after a specified time ...

You should give this to everyone with whom you live or work closely – and carry one yourself. Spend time going through it with people, and be prepared to answer or find answers to questions. Feedback can be invaluable. If anything is unclear, rewrite your plan as necessary or for an individual's benefit. Pin up customized copies at your home, place of study, or place of work. Encourage friends to carry theirs with them at all times, and don't be shy about gently performing 'spot-checks' or 'tests' of their understanding.

Emergency drills

Encourage family members and friends to test you with an emergency drill from time to time. Pick an emergency 'keyword' they can surprise you with, perhaps by phone. Go through the motions as if you were reacting severely while alone. Is your inhaler

---

Adrenaline injector pen Q&A

Q: I'm nervous about adrenaline. Are there any risks involved?
A: When used according to the instructions and in the doses recommended by your allergist or doctor, adrenaline is a safe drug. It's only potentially unsafe for those with heart conditions or when accidentally injected into a vein rather than the thigh muscle. If you are hesitant about any aspect of your allergy medication, speak to a nurse at your surgery.

Q: What if I forget my adrenaline?
A: Return home to fetch it. Consider having spare injector pens at various sites, such as your home and office.

Q: What if I suffer a reaction and don't have my adrenaline?
A: Dial 999 at once. Alert someone nearby. If you find yourself very near a pharmacy, there may be a case for seeking help there: pharmacists are now advised to help those suffering from anaphylactic responses, and can treat using an injector pen if there is one in stock. Avoid running or rushing about, though, as this can speed up the reaction.

Q: I'm pregnant. Can I use anti-allergy medication safely?
A: Anaphylactic incidents in mothers-to-be are rare. When they occur, your unborn child may be partly protected by the placenta, which produces a defensive, deactivating chemical against histamine. While using adrenaline injectors carries a small risk to the unborn child, normal recommendations are that your well-being must take priority. Seek specialist advice about your medication as soon as you discover you are expecting.

---

or adrenaline easily accessible and where it should be? Is your adrenaline within its expiry date? Is your mobile phone switched on, fully charged and functional? Do you know the exact address and postcode of your location? The procedure is useful in highlighting potential problem points you may need to address.

Although it's usually advisable to call emergency services – or possibly your doctor if you live in a remote area – when you experience anaphylaxis, there may be some circumstances where someone may need to take you to hospital for or following treatment. It's worth familiarizing yourself with the route in your area, and consider some 'dummy runs' with your partner or family members in the car.

4

Food sense

Part I: labelling and shopping

With thousands of foods now in our supermarkets, each containing as many as several dozen ingredients, the food-sensitive customer has to negotiate a potential allergic minefield. But with improved labelling practice and wider awareness of food sensitivities, the outlook is brightening.

Food labelling

Labels on pre-packaged products contain vast amounts of information, much of which many people ignore, or misunderstand, or both. As a food allergy sufferer, you cannot afford to do either.

Some information is required by law; some is optional. Compulsory information includes the food's name, its weight or volume, its use-by date, its ingredients, and the manufacturer's contact details – although there are occasional exceptions. Nutritional information is required when specific health-related claims are made – e.g. 'this is a low-fat product'.

Optional information includes serving suggestions, recipes, nutritional information (when no health claims are made) and recommended dietary guidelines. Separate statements reiterating the presence of allergens already specified in the ingredients listing (e.g. 'contains soya'), ingredients *excluded* from the product (e.g. 'free from wheat and milk'), and 'may contain' warnings are increasingly used, but remain optional.

Ingredients

The ingredients listing is arguably the most useful section. Barring a few but potentially significant exceptions, it presents all ingredients used deliberately in the product's manufacture, in descending order of weight.

Certain ingredients must be listed without exception. On 25 November 2005, an EU directive on food labelling came into operation, compelling manufacturers to indicate the presence of any of the 12 'major allergens', and most of their products, in pre-packed foods. These are:

- celery (and celeriac);
- crustaceans (e.g. crab, lobster, prawn);
- eggs;
- fish;
- gluten grains – barley, oats, rye, spelt, wheat;
- milk (including milk sugar, or lactose);
- mustard;
- nuts (e.g. almonds, cashews, walnuts);
- peanuts;
- sesame seeds;
- soya beans;
- sulphur dioxide and sulphites (at a concentration greater than 10 parts per million).

Some exemptions have been granted to derivatives of the 'big 12' which have undergone so much processing or refining that the likelihood of their inciting a reaction is tiny, because the allergenic proteins are no longer present in sufficient quantity. These include: cereal-derived sugars (such as glucose syrup) and distillates (such as whisky); fish, milk and egg products used as fining or clarifying agents in alcoholic drinks; and refined soya, mustard and celery seed oils.

Refined peanut oil, which is highly unlikely to trigger a reaction, is not exempt, however. The Anaphylaxis Campaign has expressed concern at this omission, believing that peanut-allergic people who ignorantly consume a product containing peanut oil and suffer no ill effects, but then later learn of its presence from the label, may conclude wrongly that they are no longer peanut-sensitive and so can eat other peanut products regardless.

Nevertheless, this is hugely welcome legislation, overturning the notorious '25 per cent' rule covering compound ingredients, which meant that if, for instance, the pepperoni slices on a pizza formed less than a quarter of the product's weight, the ingredients of the pepperoni did not need to be itemized, even if they included main allergens.

The ruling also demands specificity. Generic terms such as 'flavouring' now have to be replaced if the flavouring is, say, milk-derived.

Single-ingredient products, such as boxes of eggs, do not need to carry an ingredients listing. Similarly, simple dairy foods – such as cheese and yoghurt – aren't required to list 'milk' as an ingredient. Both are considered obvious.

Directive exemptions

These exemptions apply – although they are subject to review and, in several cases, the situation is expected to change in coming years, as they remain high priorities with the Food Standards Agency (FSA) and the EU.

- Possible accidental contaminants need not be declared. (But see 'May contain . . .' p. 32.)
- Loosely sold or freshly prepared food from bakeries, delicatessen counters, bars, restaurants and takeaway outlets need not be labelled.
- Other foods capable of producing allergic reactions, such as molluscs, lupin, apple and many more, must be declared unless found in one of several exempt ingredients making up less than 2 per cent of the final product. The exemptions include jams, marmalades, jellies, fruit juices, chocolate or cocoa products, spreadable fats, herb and spice mixtures and chestnut puree. So, producers of a cake containing less than 2 per cent fruit jam which includes strawberry, for instance, will not be compelled to declare the strawberry.
- Until November 2005, manufacturers of alcoholic beverages containing more than 1.2 per cent alcohol were not required to state ingredients, and although this has changed inasmuch as the 'big 12' must be declared (some distillates excepted), other potentially allergenic ingredients can still be omitted, irrespective of the quantity used.

Beware that products labelled before the 25 November 2005 cut-off point will be allowed to remain on sale until bought or passing their sell-by date. So products with long shelf-lives, such as alcoholic drinks, may remain on sale for years to come.

'Contains ...'

Many manufacturers are now voluntarily adding 'contains' boxes or statements to products, as at-a-glance references to any of the major allergens deliberately included. Useful though this is, do not base a decision about a food's safety exclusively upon it.

The FSA recommends that if a 'contains' box is present, it should mention *all* major allergens. For example, if a product declares wheat, fish and soya in its ingredients, the 'contains' box, if included, should state 'Contains wheat, fish and soya'. Beware, though, that it is not illegal for only one or two to be noted.

'May contain ...'

So-called defensive labelling – 'may contain traces of nuts', for example – is used by manufacturers for two reasons: to warn the public that a particular allergen, although not intentionally added, might have accidentally contaminated the product or its ingredients somewhere along the growing, harvesting, transporting or manufacturing line; and also to disclaim any liability in the event of a customer suffering a severe reaction because of a rogue allergen.

This declaration is not a legal requirement, but increasingly, it seems, food producers are using it – both when necessary, and also perhaps when unnecessary. Many consumers and campaigners are dismayed by this, arguing that it can be confusing to sufferers left unable to gauge the degree of risk of contamination because the message is vague and non-specific. Overzealous 'may contain' labelling also restricts food choices.

Nevertheless, cases of nut traces (and other allergens) turning up in foods carrying 'may contain' warnings are far from unknown. Improvements in policy are expected soon, as the FSA continues to work with manufacturers and other bodies. Meanwhile, always heed 'may contain' advice.

'Free from ...'

A useful piece of information, listing the major allergens which the manufacturer guarantees are absent.

If you are wheat-allergic, note that 'free from gluten' is not equivalent to 'free from wheat'. Gluten is the dominant protein found in wheat and related grains, but there are other proteins in wheat to which you may be allergic. Some products are made from wheat starch – essentially wheat stripped of its gluten – but some trace proteins can remain to which you may react.

Equally, a product labelled 'wheat-free' may still contain rye, which is a gluten grain. If you react to wheat gluten, it is likely you will also react to rye gluten. If you have been eating certain products without problem, then it is probably OK for you to continue doing so.

Other labelling information

Alternative means of conveying allergy information are used.

In 2005, Tesco implemented a five-stage warning system ranging from 'free from nuts' to 'contains nuts' on own-brand products. The three intermediate warnings are used for foods whose recipes are free from nuts, whose ingredients cannot be guaranteed nut-free, and which carry varying degrees of risk of contamination from factories or their equipment.

Elsewhere, the messages are less standardized. 'Not suitable for nut allergy sufferers' is an often-seen message – and may be used as an additional declaration of a product's nut content or, equally, as an alternative to a 'may contain' warning. Frustratingly, the reason may not be given. 'This product is manufactured in a factory where nuts are handled' is a variation, from which the degree of risk is still tough to assess. 'Prepared on equipment previously used to make products containing nuts' is another, better disclaimer, which implies a higher-risk food.

Some products carry handy 'allergy advice' sections, summarizing key information. Look out too for V symbols or 'suitable for vegetarians/vegans', which denote that products are free from fish, crustaceans, molluscs and meat, and in the case of vegan, from egg, dairy products and honey too.

Calling customer services can help answer questions; staff are now used to handling allergy queries. You can also write to manufacturers to enquire about their allergy policy. Be specific. The more we question companies in this way, the more allergy-aware they will become and the more likely they will implement improvements. Many larger firms can supply lists of guaranteed risk-free foods; some can confirm they operate nut-free sites – such as Bernard Matthews and HP Foods.

Finally, bear in mind that products in ethnic stores and delicatessens, sourced from outside the EU, may slip through, carrying insufficient, mistranslated or otherwise unclear labelling. Nuts, for instance, can be described in obscurely coded terms, such as 'fruits in shell'.

Product recalls and food alerts

Mistakes occur in food manufacturing – products can get contaminated with food allergens and find their way onto the shelf before the error is detected. When noticed, though, a food industry increasingly nervous about litigation leaps into action, and there are several ways messages will be conveyed to consumers.

Manufacturers may take out prominent advertising in national newspapers, explaining the nature of the problem, the batch number or product code of affected foods, and advice on what to do if you have bought the product. Their websites will also carry the warning, and many issue e-mail newsletters to customers – so if you rely on certain companies' products, register with them or subscribe to their bulletins.

Look out for conspicuous product-recalling signs in supermarkets, located either at checkouts, customer service counters or where the products in question are stocked.

Allergy UK and the Anaphylaxis Campaign promptly e-mail food alerts to members and their websites carry updated warnings too. The Food Standards Agency issues food alerts, including allergen alerts. You can register at: www.food. gov.uk/enforcement/alerts – or you can have alerts sent free to your mobile, by texting 'FSA' to 07866 428260.

Shopping

The bad news: shopping with a food allergy is frustrating and time-consuming. The good news: the situation is ever-improving. See 'Useful addresses' for the suppliers and manufacturers which can make your life easier.

The biggest development comes in internet shopping. Several specialist dietary suppliers now operate online, offering hundreds of products for those eating under restrictions. Buying online can spare you lengthy trawls of supermarket aisles, scrutinizing label after label – though check deliveries carefully when they arrive.

The 'free-from' market is booming, with many manufacturers specializing in niche ranges. Supermarkets and outlets such as Boots and health stores stock a range of specialist products; often you'll find sections devoted to restricted diets, including own-brand foods.

There are drawbacks to 'free-from' foods, though. First, they can be costly. Second, they're not always the healthiest of products – often, they're heavily sweetened, or processed, or they contain a host of additives. Finally, they're occasionally guilty of making an inappropriate virtue of their 'free-from' status – products proclaiming 'allergy-friendly' should be treated with caution. A wheat-free product may indeed be friendly to a wheat-allergic person, but it may also be hostile to a nut-allergic. No food is ever wholly 'allergy-friendly'; it depends entirely on the person, not the product.

Plenty of foods not specifically aimed at you will of course be suitable. Supermarkets offer fact sheets or lists of products guaranteed free from many allergens, and their customer service teams will be happy to send you them, though check their websites first. With safe foods, it is good practice to buy in bulk and freeze, saving time and money, and sparing some of the inconvenience your restrictions impose.

The golden rule remains this: carefully read the label of every item that goes into your trolley, no matter how familiar, every time you shop. Recipes and manufacturing processes change regularly, and a once safe food can become a hazard overnight. Supermarket lists date equally quickly.

The grey area remains non-pre-packed food sold at bakeries and deli-counters. Contamination is a real possibility here, simply by virtue of close storage, handling, or through a 'wandering' spoon or knife. Meat products may be sliced on machinery also used for cheeses, transferring allergens between the two. By all means enquire of staff, but it is unlikely they will be able to offer the absolute guarantee you may need.

Tree nuts and peanuts

It's wise to avoid all nuts and their products if you are allergic to any one or more, due to the risk of cross-reactions, cross-contamination on production lines, or both – unless you are certain neither presents a risk.

A reminder: as allergies in this category are potentially so serious, it is imperative you read and reread all labels. Given that research has shown as minuscule a quantity as 1/44,000th of a peanut can trigger a reaction in an exquisitely sensitive individual, any 'may-contain' warnings *must* be heeded. Typically, the culprits are found in the following foods, although this list cannot be exhaustive:

- praline, marzipan, frangipane and nougat, and some sweets, desserts, biscuits, yoghurts and chocolate products;
- vegetarian products – nut roasts and veggie burgers;
- spreads – nut butters, Nutella;
- some cereals and cereal bars;
- satays, some curries and chillis, and other sauces and marinades, especially those of east or south-east Asian origin;
- stuffings and stuffing mixes;
- some salads and salad dressings;
- unrefined nut oils or vegetable oil blends.

Tree nuts will be labelled unambiguously, but peanuts occasionally go by the names of groundnuts, monkey nuts, earth nuts, beer nuts, arachide (French/Italian) or cacahuete (Spanish), and you should also look out for peanut sprouts – used in some stir-fry mixes – which look like bean sprouts.

Because of cross-reactivity, seeds are a risk. Pine nuts (actually seeds) can be a hazard, for example; beware their use in Italian pesto sauce, as well as in other foods in which nuts are often found. Cross-reactions with coconut and nutmeg are uncommon, and in those cases the responses are usually milder. Water chestnuts are safe; chestnuts may not be.

Some additive gums are derived from obscure legumes related to peanuts – such as locust bean gum (E410), guar gum (E412), gum tragacanth (E413), acacia/arabic gum (E414) and tara gum (E417) – but the threat to peanut allergics is low. Other legumes – beans, lentils, peas – occasionally pose a problem, as do chickpeas, which can go by the names 'garbanzo', 'gram' or 'gram flour'. Vastly more dangerous is lupin (p. 42).

Those with almond allergy should avoid almond essence and also be aware of the risk of cross-reactions with apricot kernels, used to make amaretto biscuits and liqueur.

Fish, crustaceans and molluscs

These three are biologically distinct, so in theory cross-reactions should not occur between members of different groups. If you react to members of more than one group, it's likely you have distinct allergies. Cross-reactions between members of the same group are common. See Appendix 2 for a list of seafood families.

If you react to any seafood, many practitioners suggest you steer clear of all – partly because of the risk of cross-contamination at fish counters, markets, or restaurants. That said, tuna-allergics can sometimes tolerate tinned tuna, as the canning process seems to deactivate many allergens. Typical products to avoid are:

- fish-based dishes, such as paella, bouillabaisse and kedgeree;
- many Asian dishes, such as Thai or Indian fish curries;
- sauces such as fish sauce, oyster sauce, Worcestershire sauce;
- Japanese foods such as sushi, sashimi and surimi/crabstick – which may contain white fish and shellfish;
- fish pâtés and pastes, such as 'Gentleman's Relish' and potted shrimp;
- salads such as Caesar salad, tuna Niçoise or prawn cocktail;
- some stocks, soups, processed foods and ready meals;
- fish oil-fortified 'functional' foods, such as some cereal bars or milks.

Calcium and glucosamine sulphate supplements may be derived from shellfish. Vegetarian and vegan food is seafood-free; Jewish (kosher) food is shellfish-free.

Note that molluscs are not among the 'big 12' allergens.

Wheat and related gluten grains

The use of wheat is widespread, partly because of its additional role as a thickener or stabilizer. Products include:

- most flours, breads and baked products – both sweet and savoury;

- most cereals;
- most pastas, some noodles;
- processed meat and fish products – burgers, pies, sausages, pâtés and battered products like fish fingers;
- processed vegetarian products – battered vegetables, pâtés, some tinned vegetables and soups;
- some processed dairy products, such as cheese spreads, thickened milks and creams;
- drinks, including beers (usually made from barley, but sometimes wheat and more rarely rye) and instant or malt drinks;
- confectionery, including chocolate bars, sweets, chewing gum and liquorice;
- stock cubes, gravy granules, some condiments and blended seasonings.

Ingredients which can be made from wheat include cereal binder, cereal filler or cereal protein. Hydrolyzed or textured vegetable protein (HVP/TVP) may, rarely, also be made using wheat (more commonly soya), although these are less likely to pose a problem as their intense processing destroys some allergens.

Gluten is the dominant protein in wheat, and gliadin – a constituent of gluten – is a main wheat allergen. Consequently, other gluten grains – rye, barley, kamut, spelt, triticale – are prime candidates for cross-reactions. If you are gliadin-allergic, foods labelled gluten-free should be safe.

It is possible to be allergic to wheat proteins other than gliadin/ gluten. Foods labelled gluten-free are often – but not always – wheat-free, so take care.

Wheat-free products are now commonplace, though be aware of the danger of cross-reactions with other gluten grains used as wheat substitutes, especially in flours, pastas and breads. Triticale is a wheat–rye hybrid; while spelt and kamut are both types of wheat, no matter what you're told in health stores or by specialist manufacturers of wheat-free products.

Although most beers are made from barley not wheat (some German and Belgian beers being exceptions), cross-contamination or cross-reactions may be an issue. Some manufacturers are now producing wheat- and gluten-free beers. However, the Institute of Food Research thinks beer allergy can be distinct from cereal allergy, as its proteins are highly modified, and has suggested a link to peach allergy, common in the Mediterranean.

If you can tolerate rye, then pumpernickel, rye crackers and rye flakes are excellent alternatives – but ensure all products' wheat-free status first.

Oats are also gluten grains, but are more removed from other family members, and so cross-reactions are less likely. You may be able to tolerate oats if you're allergic to other gluten cereals. Check products such as oatcakes carefully to ensure wheat flour has not been added.

Dairy food

Obvious products here are milk, cheese, cream, yoghurt, ice cream and butter.

A few dairy-allergics may find they can tolerate UHT, evaporated or condensed milks, and traces of milk found in some ready meals which have undergone a lot of processing. If you have been eating certain products without problem since your milk allergy diagnosis, it is generally considered OK for you to carry on. Always exercise caution, though, and check with your consultant.

Vigilance is necessary, as milk products turn up in an array of foods:

- sweet baked products, such as cakes, pancakes and biscuits;
- savoury baked goods, such as breads (in America), crisps and crackers;
- sweets and confectionery, including most chocolate;
- ready meals, processed meats, convenience products;
- soups – typically 'cream of' soups;
- dips, spreads, dressings, gravies and sauces;
- cereals and snack bars;
- instant hot drinks and cream liqueurs;
- some sweeteners.

Terms denoting milk extracts include casein, caseinate, curds and whey. The lactate additives (E325–9) and the sugar lactitol (E966) are generally milk-derived but are unlikely to affect you.

Look for vegan foods and those labelled dairy-free. There are several 'cheeses' and 'yoghurts' available, generally made from soya, as well as many 'milks' made from nuts, legumes, grains and tubers.

Cream of tartar and cocoa butter are dairy-free.

Eggs

Allergy to egg white is more common than to yolk, but as cross-contamination cannot be guaranteed against, and labelling may not be specific, it is safer to steer clear of all egg-containing products if you're allergic. Aside from obvious sources – quiches, omelettes, mayonnaises – many prepared foods also contain egg:

- egg noodles, fresh pastas and sauces (e.g. carbonara);
- many baked goods, such as biscuits, buns, pastries and cakes – often as a glaze, for instance on bagels and pretzels;
- processed breaded or battered foods;
- dressings and sauces (e.g. Hollandaise, tartare);
- desserts – custard, mousse, meringue, crème caramel;
- icing, and confectionery – again possibly as a glaze;
- Advocaat liqueur;
- surimi/crabsticks.

The additive lecithin (E322), although usually soya-derived, is very occasionally produced from yolk.

Egg replacers or substitutes, available from health-food shops, are useful for cooking, but some may contain egg whites. Choose vegan egg replacers.

Soya

Used abundantly in Chinese and Japanese cuisines, soya is widely employed here as a milk, protein and meat alternative, and its flour as a wheat flour replacement. It is found in many foods, especially convenience foods, and so is tough to avoid. These are a few examples:

- most vegan/vegetarian burgers, pies, sausages, pâtés and prepared meals, and many meat equivalents;
- soya milks, 'cheeses' and 'yoghurts';
- many other specialist dietetic products, such as gluten-free foods;
- some cakes, biscuits, pastries and confectionery;

- fermented soya products, such as soy sauce, tofu, tempeh and miso;
- many infant food formulas;
- any prepared food labelled hydrolyzed or textured vegetable proteins (HVP/TVP – usually soya), vegetable starch or gum (also often soya), soya caseinate, lecithin (E322) and monosodium glutamate (MSG/E621 – often a soya processing by-product).

Sesame and other seeds

Sesame is found in the Mediterranean and Middle Eastern foods houmous, halva and tahini, and widely in Chinese and other Asian cuisines.

There are many alternative names for it which may crop up on imported products, including ajonjoli (Spain/South America), benne/benniseed (West Africa), cingili/gingelly (India), simsim (East Africa) and teel/til (Asia).

Seeds such as sesame, poppy, pumpkin and sunflower – which can cross-react with each other and with nuts – are increasingly used in a variety of products, sometimes unexpectedly:

- baked goods, such as speciality breads, burger buns, biscuits, crackers and cakes, often as decoration, and any unwrapped or loose bakery products, which may be contaminated;
- many prepared meals, such as burgers, vegeburgers, sausages, curries and nut roasts;
- cereals and cereal snack bars;
- unrefined seed oils – such as sesame oil, Chinese stir-fry oils or oils used in salad dressings – and spreads (sunflower spread);
- spice mixtures, such as gomashio (Japanese sesame salt);
- lecithin (E322) – occasionally sunflower-derived.

Mustard

Beware condiments such as chutneys or pickles, flavourings, spice mixtures or prepared salad dressings. Mustard and cress seedlings don't need to be labelled as they're not pre-packed, but according to the FSA, 'much of what is sold as "cress" in the UK comes from other plants and doesn't include any mustard'. Be alert to the risk of cross-reactions, though.

Celery

Found in Waldorf salad (and perhaps other prepared salads), many vegetable stocks or stock cubes, the rice dish jambalaya, in celery spice and other seasonings, in many Italian tomato-based pasta sauces and in health tonics such as 'detox' juices.

Lupin

Not on the list of major food allergens – and considered one of the most dangerous omissions in light of its capacity to cross-react with peanut.

Commonly used in France and neighbouring countries, high-protein sweet lupin is becoming popular as a soya replacement, and its flour is used in imported bakery, pastries, pastas and other catering, fast-food products, such as meat, fish or vegetable batters. Sometimes it shows up unexpectedly in cereals, snack bars, and chocolate or carob confectionery.

Corn/maize

Corn allergy is principally a North American problem. Obvious sources such as sweetcorn, corn flakes, other cereals and Italian polenta aside, products to check include:

- ready meals, soups and sauces;
- ready made desserts and confectionery;
- tortilla wraps and chips, tacos and other convenience snacks;
- baked goods, especially specialist gluten-free products;
- some baking powders;
- any label reading vegetable protein, or hydrolyzed or textured vegetable protein (HVP/TVP – occasionally corn-derived);
- any label reading edible starch, food starch, modified starch, vegetable starch, cereal starch, glucose syrup (all may be corn-derived), corn syrup, maltodextrin or dextrose – though the risk is low.

Meat

Allergy to meat is rare, and thorough cooking destroys many of its allergens. It is easy to avoid. Cross-reactions between egg, chicken and turkey are possible. Reactions to processed meat products may be due to added milk, soya or wheat – these are all used widely in foods such as sausages, pies and burgers.

Tomatoes

Found in many prepared products. Check all pasta sauces, red-coloured pasta, chillies, pizzas, curries, condiments (chutneys, ketchups), baked beans and other tinned foods, concentrates, soups, salads and juices.

In those with OAS-related tomato allergy, only raw tomatoes seem to pose a problem – usually the riper the tomato, the worse the reaction.

Mushrooms and fungi

Mushrooms are found in some prepared meals, stir-fries and salads, and in some sauces, flavourings and stock cubes. Cross-reactions with related foods such as truffles and mycoprotein or Quorn – made from a form of fungus – are possible.

Other vegetables

Reactions to cooked vegetables are rare, but if you experience any you will need to scrutinize labelling on all prepared meals, foods and products such as soups and stock cubes.

Raw vegetable juices are increasingly used in juice blends, and of course raw vegetables will be found in prepared salads.

Alcoholic beverages and aperitifs, and health or 'detox' tonics often contain vegetable extracts. Some of these are surprising. In particular members of the daisy family, including artichoke, dandelion, echinacea and milk thistle are used in many concoctions. Those with OAS to mugwort or ragweed – which can cross-react with daisy family members – should take care.

Fruits

Depending on your allergies, and whether or not you only react to the raw fruit, you may need to check items such as fruit salads, jams, chutneys and other condiments, fruit vinegars (and salad dressings), desserts, chocolates and confectionery, cereals and cereal bars, herbal and fruit teas, and even ready meals.

Take especial care with juice blends, as the name of the product may only mention one or two fruits, yet the ingredients may show the presence of others.

The same goes for spirits, many of which are flavoured with fruits, such as Calvados (apple) and Cointreau (orange), and so-called alcopop drinks, which may have many fruity additions.

Those with apple allergy should check for the carbohydrate pectin (E440), derived from apples (or sometimes orange), and used as a setting agent, for instance in jams, in which trace allergens might be found. Apple juices – and sometimes other fruit juices – are also used as sweeteners, often in sugar-free products, dairy-free milks and sometimes products such as soups.

For those with fruit allergies related to OAS, most of these are unlikely to pose problems; only the raw fruits and freshly squeezed fruit juices are of concern, usually. Organic, freshly picked or under-ripe fruit may be marginally less reactive.

The allergenic proteins responsible for mild oral reactions tend to be destroyed by pasteurization and processing – so juices made from concentrates or stored in cartons outside the chiller cabinet will probably be safe. Similarly, you should be OK with tinned fruit.

Unexpected ingredients

The importance of reading labels when shopping is perhaps best emphasized by some examples of unexpected ingredients. These aren't intended to alarm you, merely to alert you to the care you need to take.

- Lea & Perrins Worcestershire sauce contains *anchovy*;
- Bombay Sapphire gin contains *almonds*;
- Italian Mortadella ham contains *pistachios*;
- Aqua Libra drink contains *sesame* and *sunflower*;
- Marmite contains *celery*;
- Branston Pickle contains *rice*;
- Wrigley's Extra gum contains *soya*;
- Jacob's cream crackers contain *egg*;
- Salute gluten-free pasta fusili contain *lupin*.

Herbs and spices

Again, allergies to these are uncommon, and usually related to OAS. In small amounts, herbs and spices may be hidden on labels under generic terms such as 'flavourings', 'spices' or 'curry powder', for instance. Check ready meals, spice mixtures, stock cubes, condiments, salad dressings, herbal teas and health tonics.

Part II: cooking and eating

Preventing reactions – by avoiding your food allergens – is the cornerstone of good food-allergy management. To succeed, you must make sure every bite of food you eat is safe. Sadly, as you may already know from experience, this is a formidable task.

Ready-prepared foods

Ideally, any pre-packed or prepared foods or meals to which you may react will remain on supermarket shelves and never accompany you to the checkout. In practice, oversights happen when you're rushed, and potentially troublesome foods can end up in your shopping basket and your kitchen.

So, before you use any foods in your larder, recheck labels. It takes seconds, and could spare you a reaction. Besides, if a partner or flatmate has done the shopping, you may be examining a product for the first time.

Many foods – especially 'bumper' boxes or multi-packs – come in extra layers of wrapping, so once you've read outer labelling, ensure you read labels on the individual items inside too. There have been cases where external and internal details have not tallied. If you ever find a discrepancy, report it to the manufacturer and the allergy charities.

Also, scrutinize the food itself. Does it look like the product described on the label? Very rarely packaging errors occur when products end up carrying the wrong sleeves or labelling information.

Cooking

The main advantages of home cooking are that you can control what goes into your meals and be confident of those meals being safe and wholesome.

Cooking for yourself is also grounding and relaxing, can make you more 'food-aware', and cultivates a healthier relationship with food – one where you look upon it as something to be enjoyed and savoured, not as a potential enemy. From a health perspective, freshly prepared meals based on unprocessed ingredients are likely to provide better nutrition. It can be more time-consuming, granted, but to compensate you'll need to devote less time to reading labels.

There are many cookbooks on the market aimed at people on restricted diets – such as dairy-free, wheat-free, egg-free, corn-free and more. The internet is a good means of tracking down titles; try searching for 'allergy eating' or 'cooking egg-free', for example. Antoinette Savill, Barbara Cousins, Michelle Berriedale-Johnson and Rita Greer are some writers to look out for. Endeavour to find one devoted to your specific allergy, rather than an 'all-purpose' cookbook which excludes foods to which you may not react. Vegetarian and vegan books are also filled with imaginative ideas, as are magazines such as *Foods Matter* and *Allergy*.

Denaturing food

Cooking some foods, and so breaking down their trigger proteins, can make them safe – for some people.

Those more likely to benefit are those living with OAS. Cooking the fruits, vegetables and herbs implicated in OAS usually makes them safe – although be aware this is far less likely if you experience reactions to raw foods not connected to hay fever.

The more fibrous a fruit or vegetable is, the more cooking it is likely to need to thoroughly deactivate its allergens. This does not mean, though, that you should cook all vegetables into a pulp, but that some cautious experimentation with cooking times is advised to establish tolerance thresholds. Boiling, steaming, microwaving and roasting are all effective; but flash- or stir-frying, although very hot, may not denature all allergens if cooking times are short.

Peeling can sometimes make a fruit safe or less reactive. Those with mild apple allergies related to hay fever sometimes find this, because many apple allergens are concentrated under the skin.

However, food preparation itself is not without minor hazards. It is often advisable to ask someone to peel vegetables for you or to wear cooking gloves or a face mask. Closely handling foods to which you react – peeling, slicing or chopping them, for instance – is likely to trigger rashes on your hands, aggravate your eyes and nose, and possibly make you wheezy if you inhale vapours. Cooking vapours – generally from boiling or frying – can also trigger asthma-like symptoms.

Cooking will not denature all allergens, though. Many still react to some spices, and to celery. In one study of patients testing positive for celery and birch or mugwort pollens, 94 per cent reacted positively to raw celery, but 36 per cent still reacted to cooked celery.

Cooking will have little or no beneficial effect on seeds and nuts, which are best avoided if you react to them.

Latex–food cross-reactions

The allergenic proteins found in tropical fruits and other foods implicated in cross-reactions with latex allergy are hardier than those found in fruit and vegetables connected to pollen sensitivities. More intense and prolonged cooking is likely to be required to remove or reduce the possibility of a reaction, although in many cases heat will have no effect.

Cooked potato, for example, is usually well tolerated, as is cooked banana. The allergens in chestnut and avocado, though, resist heat treatment. However, everyone reacts differently, so exercise caution unless you are certain a food is safe.

Other foods

In general, those reacting to the major allergenic foods need to avoid all forms of their triggers.

It is impossible to cover all permutations, but there can be exceptions. Cooking can alter the allergenicity of both fish and egg, both for the better and worse, depending on the individual.

If you have been consuming a particular food or product cooked or processed in a certain way with no problem since your diagnosis, then it is generally considered safe to assume you may carry on doing so. Beware, though, of complacency: should you react to raw egg but not cooked, for instance, a speedily prepared omelette when you're running late can have consequences.

Replacement ingredients

Milk: try natural coconut milk in sweet recipes, or in hot drinks or on cereal try any of the range of other alternative 'milks' now widely available, including soya, oat, almond, hazelnut and potato.

Cheese: tofu, soya 'cheeses'.

Cream: creamed coconut or other nuts pasted and blended with warm water and maybe honey.

Yoghurt: soya yoghurts or desserts; for dressings or dips, experiment with plain mayonnaise.

Wheat flour: for baking, try a mix of other flours – such as rye, oat, buckwheat and potato – combined with either guar or xanthan gums to prevent crumbling. For thickening, corn-starch, tapioca or arrowroot are good.

Pasta: rice noodles, buckwheat noodles (soba) or corn pasta.

Cereal grains: try buckwheat (not a true wheat), quinoa, amaranth.

Egg: for glazing, try a honey or sugar solution, or gelatine (also a useful setting agent); for binding, try pureed banana or apple, tofu or a soya dessert; for leavening, use baking powder and some liquid.

Nuts and seeds: As a snack, popcorn or other popped grains; fried croutons to add 'crunch' to salads.

Cooking and eating at home

Most people adapt easily to the changes required by a diagnosis of food allergy, and quickly establish workable routines. So will you. Here are some tips which may help:

- wash (or peel) all fresh produce that may have come into contact with other people or foods – allergen traces can spread easily;
- get organized with menu planning: it helps to dictate efficient weekly shopping and avoid last-minute what-to-cook dilemmas;
- cook safe sauces and soups and other staples in large quantities, and freeze batches, so that you always have allergy-safe home-cooked meals available when you come home tired and hungry, or to feed allergic family members, all at short notice;

- have safe ready-to-eat snacks in cupboards too, in case you really can't wait;
- never reuse oils in which you've previously cooked unsafe foods;
- guard against absent-minded sampling of food if you're cooking for family members who don't share your allergy – chewing a piece of gum can help;
- in large households, take care with cross-contamination – traces of dairy spreads in the jam jar, wheaten toast crumbs in the butter tray – and encourage everyone to use separate items of cutlery for each food;
- have separate utensils for cooking allergen-friendly and non-allergen-friendly foods, and closely examine them to ensure they're spotless before use;
- if you try new foods, check the food families they or their ingredients belong to first, so you can identify any potential cross-reactors; only ever do so when you are not alone, have your medication, and are close to a phone; and preferably try them in the morning or early afternoon when you're more likely to be alert to any possible reaction and less likely to have had alcohol;
- store allergic foods separately – in plastic containers in the fridge for instance – and where they can't contaminate or be contaminated by other foods – such as by a leaking milk carton;
- aim to keep a clean, tidy, hygienic kitchen, as good kitchen management will guard against slip-ups – wash cupboards, refrigerators and worktops regularly;
- in the case of serious allergies within a large household, consider imposing a total ban on the food in question – as do most families with a nut-allergic member – and ensure everyone, visitors included, understands the rule.

Eating out

Most serious food allergic reactions occur away from the home and are caused by food prepared by others.

Yet eating out is probably an important part of your social life and you should not deny yourself this pleasure; instead, make plans and take every precaution possible to ensure your safety and enjoyment.

Where to eat

Choose restaurants whose cuisines are unlikely to trouble you. Asian restaurants – Thai, Chinese, Malaysian – are good choices for wheat- and dairy-allergics, for example, but not good for fish- or nut-allergics. Ask fellow allergics for recommendations. Share your problem with friends and colleagues: avoiding a particular restaurant is not awkward if everyone knows of your condition.

Call ahead if you plan to eat at a restaurant to ask whether you can be catered for. If your condition is life-threatening, emphasize it in clear terms. Be direct with questioning. Be prepared for the person taking your call to put you on hold to check with chefs. If ultimately they sound doubtful, don't book the table.

If you intend dining at one of a chain of high street restaurants, it's worth searching its website or calling its customer services helpline to find out its policy on food allergy. Some are excellent in this respect, and can let you know which meals, the ingredients of which are often standardized, should be safe.

Eating or drinking at an independent café, takeaway outlet, bar or pub can be riskier, because quality control is unlikely to be as stringent and ingredient lists may not be available; since food and meals are unlikely to have been prepared on site, reassurances may not be absolute.

Be aware that you can be exposed to allergens in surprising ways: foamed eggs are occasionally used as toppings on coffee or other bar drinks and foods at self-service areas can easily be cross-contaminated by wandering cutlery. If the chef has used latex gloves in preparing food, traces of milk proteins – used in latex glove manufacture – can transfer to food and trigger a reaction in dairy allergics.

The websites www.harid.co.uk and www.foodfreefrom.co.uk offer searchable directories of recommended eateries; www.veggie heaven.com has one of vegetarian and vegan restaurants.

Ordering

When you arrive at a restaurant which you haven't pre-booked, make sure you inform a member of staff immediately about your allergy. Ask if they can check whether there are safe foods available. Don't be shy of articulating the precise consequences of contamination or errors. Ensure your conversation is witnessed by members of your party. If you are not confident the gravity of your condition is appreciated, don't eat there.

Read menus carefully. Never let hunger or impatience get the better of judgement. Ask waiting staff to clarify ambiguities and specify safe meals – possibly recommended by the chefs. If you can speak to a chef, so much the better; you'll be able to better gauge their degree of confidence in the meal they're serving you.

Don't be shy of questioning staff; they are now accustomed to hearing specific dietary needs and can be increasingly relied upon to convey those stipulations accurately to kitchen staff. Is the chef 100 per cent certain of all the ingredients he uses in his recipe? Might a food be cooked in oil previously used to cook a risk food, such as fish? Are separate utensils, chopping boards and knives used to prepare different foods? What are the ingredients of the salad dressings? Have the 'safe' desserts been stored alongside nut-containing desserts? Listen carefully to the replies given.

Do this even in restaurants in which you've previously dined and which have come to 'know' you. Never become complacent. Suppliers, ingredients, chefs, recipes and menus all change. Always check, every time.

People living with OAS are better off ordering cooked food, which ensures any allergens have been denatured by heat. Some people with latex–food allergy may be able to get away with a similar tactic, but the most sensitive need to take greater care: even the use of latex gloves in the kitchen can leave rubber traces on food to which you may react. Note too that potentially cross-reacting enzymic fruits – such as mango, pineapple, papaya and kiwi – are sometimes used by chefs to tenderize meat.

Understandably, there will be times when you may not want to go through this rigmarole. A bit depressing, perhaps, but in this instance plain food is often safest – like meat and vegetables, or a baked potato and cheese. Soups, stews, pies and other dishes where ingredients are disguised or hidden are best avoided.

Precautions

Your fellow diners should know about your allergy and about the consequences of your consuming your trigger allergens. Ensure someone has a copy of your emergency action plan (see p. 26) and knows where your medication is kept.

When your food arrives, use your eyes and nose. Does it look and smell as if it is free from your trigger? Ask someone to taste it if you need to, and start off cautiously. Send back anything you're suspicious of. Never pick allergens out of food you are served – especially nut toppings off desserts. Reconfirm with waiting staff that your meal is safe: in busy restaurants, with many clients to attend to, instructions can be forgotten and mistakes made.

And finally ...

Make a point at the end of the meal of thanking staff for catering for you. It will encourage them to become more allergy-aware. Further, spread the word and report excellent establishments to others in similar situations, charities and relevant bodies.

Visiting friends

Being invited to dinner and having to inform your hosts of your allergy can feel awkward, but you must impress upon them the seriousness of your condition. Ease your discomfort by offering to help with the preparations and cooking, or to bring your own safe ingredients or dishes.

Buffets and parties are more problematic, as food arrangements here can be more cavalier. Be wary of cross-contamination issues, and guard against absent-minded nibbling while you're busy socializing. Cocktail snacks like sushi and Chinese bites often have hidden egg and nut.

During national holidays or other festivities, there will be more food around, possibly alcohol, and in the buzz of celebration it is easy for hosts and those with allergies alike to forget about them. Christmas can be a hazardous time, as nuts are everywhere – in Christmas puddings, stuffings, mince pies, chocolate Brazils, dried fruit and nut mixes and so on. Be on your guard.

5

Practical issues

Although becoming 'food sensible' is an important skill to acquire in order to effectively manage your allergy, it's inevitable that other aspects of your life will need attention too.

Personal hygiene

Every day we wash, scrub, cleanse, moisturize, deodorize, condition and colour parts of our body with a boggling selection of gels, soaps, sprays, creams, pastes, unguents, powders, scents and dyes – but what of the safety of the ingredients in these potions?

Cosmetics are big business. In the fierce battle for consumer appeal, beauty and grooming companies are now placing greater emphasis on natural products – a vogue which has resulted in more grains, fruits and other botanicals finding their way into toiletries, many of them in unadulterated states, and therefore potentially more allergenic.

So what's the risk? One might think small. Personal care products are not meant for consumption and, barring lipsticks, toothpastes and mouth washes, are not used orally.

However, when you consider that shower gel can get into eyes, bath oils and scents may be inhaled, and around 60 per cent of the make-up, deodorants and creams we apply to our bodies is absorbed through the skin into the bloodstream, the picture becomes more worrying.

Product labelling

Although only food (not cosmetic items) is bound by the November 2005 directive, by law ingredients must be listed on personal care products – either on the container or the packaging. Cosmetics which are small and difficult to label clearly are partially exempt; instead, their ingredients should be displayed close to the item's point of sale or be available on a leaflet.

That said, three issues remain awkward for the consumer: botanicals are often in Latin not English (see list in box on p. 54);

the names may refer to any part of the plant – flesh, seed, shell, bark or leaf – and it might not always be clear what has been used; and the widespread use of the word 'parfum' (perfume), as a catch-all for any combination of fragrances.

Latin names of food allergens in cosmetics

Almond – prunus [amygdalus] dulcis/amara/sativa
Apple – malus domestica/pyrus malus
Apricot – prunus armeniaca
Avocado – persea gratissima/americana
Banana – musa sapientum
Barley – hordeum/hordeum vulgare
Brazil nut – bertholletia excelsa
Cashew – anacardium occidentale
Celery/celeriac – apium graveolens
Chestnut – castanea sativa/sylva
Corn – zea mays
Egg – ovum
Fish/fish oil – pisces/piscum iecur
Hazelnut – corylus rostrata/avellana
Kiwi fruit – actinidia chinensis
Lupin – lupinus albus/luteus
Macadamia nut – macadamia ternifolia
Milk – lac
Oat – avena sativa
Peach – prunus persica
Peanut – arachis/arachis hypogea
Pistachio – pistacia vera
Rice – oryza/oryza sativa
Sesame – sesamum indicum
Soya – glycine max/soja
Sunflower – helianthus annuus
Walnut – juglans regia/nigra
Wheat – triticum/triticum vulgare

Nut derivatives are sometimes used. Peanut goes by the name *arachis hypogea* and peanut oil by *arachis oil*; both can crop up in products such as soaps, make-up and emollients. They were once more common in creams – such as eczema, nipple or vaginal creams – but because of the risk of sensitizations or reactions, this is now rare. Still, always check labels. It's safer to avoid nut-containing cosmetics if your family is atopic. The same applies, clearly, if you are already sensitized, although only traces of allergen are likely to be present in the case of nut oils, and any reaction will probably be mild and localized.

Fruit kernels are sometimes used too, and these have the potential to cross-react with nuts – especially apricot or peach kernels and almonds, which belong to the same family, the rose stone or plum family, or *prunus* in Latin.

Grains and nuts tend to crop up in products of a thicker consistency, such as gels, creams and exfoliating washes, and fruits are often found in liquid shower gels and shampoos, for instance. Unexpected ingredients are more widespread in cosmetics than in foods – deodorants containing wheat protein, aftershaves containing sesame, and many more curious examples abound.

The notation [+/- ...] indicates that the ingredient(s) listed in square brackets may or may not be present – the cosmetic equivalent of a 'may contain'.

The Cosmetic Toiletry and Perfumery Association website (www.ctpa.org.uk) has more information.

Other reactions to cosmetics

Contact dermatitis, characterized by red itchy patches of skin, is the most common reaction. It is usually non-allergic and triggered by an irritant such as an abrasive or a detergent. The reaction is delayed not immediate, localized to the site of application, and usually caused by repeated exposure to the cosmetic, rather than one-off use. Eczema sufferers and very light-skinned people are more susceptible, but irritant contact dermatitis can affect anybody.

Genuine allergic contact dermatitis is less common. It is often caused by one or more of the many thousand fragrances found in body-care products, but also by preservatives, UV filters and emulsifiers. Unlike irritant contact dermatitis, allergic contact dermatitis can spread beyond the site of application. Patch testing by a dermatologist can help identify culprits. Around 2 per cent of the population may be allergic to at least one cosmetic ingredient; and people prone to other allergies, including food allergies, are more susceptible.

Immediate urticarial rashes are occasionally reported too, as are 'burns' to assorted substances. Tragically, very rarely, anaphylactic deaths have occurred due to exposure to chemical hair dyes.

Cosmetic safety

Read all labels on products, for both ingredients and instructions, and perform a patch test if recommended.

Some botanical extracts in cosmetics have the potential to cross-react with allergens to which you are already sensitized – see Appendix 2 for guidance on identifying plants which may pose problems.

Check the safety of products used by your hairdresser, beautician or even massage therapist. If you are severely reactive, avoid bathing or grooming when alone at home, or behind a locked door.

If dermatitis is a concern, avoid certain products for short periods to see whether symptoms alleviate. Don't stick to favourites: rotate safe products to avoid risking sensitization through continued use. Don't use products on broken skin. Hypoallergenic products are free from fragrances and deemed less likely to cause reactions, but there are no guarantees. The expression 'dermatologically tested' is largely meaningless.

For further advice, try the National Eczema Society Helpline (0870 241 3604), ask your doctor for a referral to a dermatologist, call Allergy UK's chemical sensitivity helpline or see the British Association of Dermatologists' website at www.bad.org.uk.

Domestic issues

Your home should be your safe haven, but when dealing with allergies you must guard against complacency. Although exposure to toiletries perhaps poses the greatest risk of a non-food reaction, there are other sources of potential triggers.

Pets

Animals can cause allergies, particularly the sweat and saliva of cats and dogs, while your pet's skin, hair and waste products may trigger asthmatic symptoms. However, as a food-allergic individual you should perhaps be more concerned with what you feed your pet.

Petfood can contain key allergens. Ingredients are typically declared on the label, although 2005's EU Directive does not apply to animal food. Dog food may have cereal grains and milk; cat food often contains fish, crustaceans, molluscs and occasionally grains; bird food may have seeds and cereals as well as milk and egg derivatives; and fish food might contain fish, crustacean, molluscan, cereal and egg derivatives.

Handling food may trigger reactions if you're sensitively allergic. Wear gloves, and take care with opening tins and packets. Keep all pet bowls and cutlery used to dispense petfood separate from domestic crockery. Dogs are messy eaters, and their food can travel across floors and be deposited on furniture only to end up on hands and be transferred to the mouth; clean up regularly and keep alert. You may need to discourage your affectionate pet from licking you enthusiastically after a feed too. If you can house or feed your pet outside the home, for instance in a designated garden or shed area, so much the better.

Household cleaning

Products such as polishes, air fresheners, washing liquids and powders, bleaches and detergents sometimes contain plant extracts, but any reactions you experience to them are likely to be chemical sensitivities not allergies.

Some of these products, and others such as aromatic candles, will also have one or more potentially allergenic fragrances, of the sort used in cosmetic products. Ingredients are rarely provided, so call manufacturers, and see your doctor if you experience responses.

Gloves and masks help minimize contact while cleaning, but it's a good idea generally to try to reduce your chemical exposures inside the home, as they can challenge the body and the immune system: why not throw open the windows instead of using air freshener, or try damp cloths not furniture sprays to wipe surfaces? Allergy UK's website has advice on keeping your home allergen-free, particularly useful if you have dust-mite allergies, or call their chemical sensitivity helpline.

Gardening

Asthma or hay fever sufferers are susceptible to pollen, spores, mould and fragrances from the garden, but you can take steps to reduce exposure. Insect-pollinated plants, such as most flowers, are safer to those liable to hay fever than wind-pollinated plants, such as trees or grasses. Avoid sniffing potently fragranced flowers, though, and ask someone else to mow the lawn. Wear gardening clothes, sunglasses, a hat and gloves to protect yourself from pollen. Asthma UK can advise further.

Members of the daisy family – including chrysanthemums, dahlias, dandelions, marigolds and feverfew – can be problematic to all those with allergies too. Handling them may cause dermatitic reactions, and they can also cross-react with other, commonly eaten members of the daisy family, such as sunflower and camomile. Take care if you have mugwort or ragweed pollen sensitivity.

Fertilizers, plant sprays, insecticides and plant foods can trigger chemical and allergic sensitivities, so protect yourself when handling them. Organic gardening products are more likely to contain plant-derived materials such as rape, soya and sunflower, so be aware of possible cross-reactions.

Finally, don't grow any plants which may trigger allergies in the family. For instance, avoid sweet lupins or perhaps other legumes if there's a risk of your peanut-allergic child coming into contact with them when playing in the garden.

Your social and personal life

You must take care in places other than food outlets and restaurants.

In pubs and bars, and with regard to drinks, provided you're certain of their ingredients, pre-bottled varieties are generally safer than draught drinks or any drinks served in glasses which may not have been scrupulously washed. Bar snacks – typically nuts – are a bigger problem, though, if you're especially sensitive, as allergens can become airborne when other drinkers are consuming them, and this can trigger a reaction. Remember alcohol clouds your judgement, slows your response and may hasten a reaction.

In clubs, the mix of dancing, loud noise and alcohol is potentially even more distracting, although there are usually fewer bar snacks. Taking recreational drugs in these situations must be avoided, as some – especially in club atmospheres – can make you paranoid, depressed or panicky, all of which could compromise your safety and lead you to use medication inappropriately.

At the cinema, many people like to eat snacks such as nuts and popcorn, and sometimes the air can get thick with food aromas. If you're highly sensitive to these allergens, ask to be seated in a secluded area, or a facial mask may help. Check seats carefully for discarded food.

If you like to get amidst a large body of people – such as at a rock concert – it's better to stick to nothing but water. Getting out of a dense crowd swiftly to access emergency treatment could be impossible in such a situation.

Many are increasingly using gyms, both to keep fit, but also as a means of getting out and socializing. If you carry medication or are susceptible to exercise-induced anaphylaxis, you must make senior people at the club and any medical staff such as first-aiders or physiotherapists aware of your condition, and always have a training buddy with you. It's worth checking that equipment is clean before you use it. Bear in mind that calorific foods such as milk protein drinks, cereal bars and nut snacks are commonly eaten by keep-fit enthusiasts to keep energy levels high, so are likely to be a constant presence.

Finally, it's worth inputting an emergency contact into your mobile phone under ICE (In Case of Emergency): useful should you have an attack, not only while out on your own, but also should you get separated from responsible friends.

Personal relationships

Kissing a relative stranger who happens to have been eating nuts or fish that day could be risky. Embarrassing, but ask before you pucker up. If you're shy, try to introduce some light humour – but ensure the seriousness of your allergy is understood by your Romeo or Juliet.

Food-allergic people report constantly how supportive partners can be to their condition, and yours will almost certainly be no exception. If you need them to sacrifice a food, they surely will.

Another point for dairy-allergics: some condoms are manufactured using a process employing the milk protein casein. Vegan condoms, such as those by Condomi, are safe.

Your professional life

If you're pondering a career in the catering or food industries, it could prove difficult to protect yourself from allergens, and employers may be reluctant to take you on. Food allergies may constitute complicating factors in other jobs too – such as caring or nursing, or piloting or airline cabin work.

If as a newly diagnosed food-allergic you already work with food, gloves and face masks might help, but may prove impractical. If you can no longer do your job, your employer has a duty to offer alternative, safer work.

Whatever your job, you must inform your employers of your condition. Large companies will have personnel departments – which can prove supportive and perhaps put you in touch with other allergic employees – as well as designated first-aid officers, whom you should train in adrenaline administration. Do likewise with close working colleagues, and consider pinning up emergency action plans (see p. 26) on noticeboards or in staff canteens.

Student life

When you combine youthful irresponsibility with the freedom of life away from home and the thrill of forging new relationships and friendships, it's perhaps only to be expected that food-allergy prevention tactics may get shunted down the list of priorities in a young person's mind.

Parents can go a long way to remind their young charges of their responsibilities to look after themselves. Urge them to take an interest in their condition, join relevant groups, and read widely on the subject. It's also worth pre-emptively 'training' adolescents for the prospect of flying the nest: for instance, by encouraging them even as young children to order their own food in restaurants and explain their allergies to waiting staff, rather than you doing it for them. The Anaphylaxis Campaign runs regular workshops for teens which can help prepare them for future independence, and also publishes a guidance booklet.

As a student, it's important you get used to the implications of fending for yourself and take responsibility for carrying your medication at all times. With regard to further education, you should be sent a questionnaire by the admissions tutor once acceptance is confirmed, on which you should declare your allergy. Many colleges and universities can cater well for those on limited diets – perhaps by teaming you up with flatmates with similar restrictions in self-catering, or by guaranteeing nut-free meals at least once a day. The sooner you let them know, the more likely they will be able to arrange help.

When there, those who need to know of your allergy include close fellow students, the college nurse, your new doctor, your hall of residence warden, the catering manager, your tutors and any university first-aiders. Speak to university medical staff about your condition, and the best procedure in the event of an emergency. You may need to adjust your emergency action plan accordingly. Don't forget to give one to friends, tutors and wardens, perhaps with a clear photograph of you attached. Pin some up on visible notice-boards too.

Larger universities may have student allergy support societies. If there isn't one where you're studying, form one: a terrific way of meeting people in the same boat as you and setting up a network of young people always on the lookout for one another.

Medicine and healthcare

Unfortunately, a lot of medicines are manufactured using allergenic foods, including wheat, soya, corn and egg. Dairy is used regularly in medicines and tablets (including oral contraceptives), and even sesame or peanut oil crop up occasionally in pharmaceuticals. Many joint supplements, such as glucosamine and those containing essential omega oils, may be derived from shellfish and fish respectively.

Every time you are prescribed medication remind your doctor of your allergy. When you collect it from the pharmacist, confirm that it is free of your trigger. Read labels and instructions – not just for allergens, but also for any possible interactions with your allergy medication. This applies to inhalants, topical creams and any medicines taken internally.

Do the same with over-the-counter medication or supplements; it's always worth enquiring whether allergy-free alternatives are available.

Inform and remind all healthcare workers – dentists, chiropodists, physical therapists – of your allergy before they treat you.

Wearing personalized medical-alert necklets or bracelets such as those offered by the charity MedicAlert is recommended should you be at risk of anaphylaxis or any other condition which may require emergency treatment, either here or abroad.

Vaccinations

Influenza and yellow fever vaccines are cultured on egg, and pose a potential risk to extremely sensitive egg-allergics, should trace proteins be present in the vaccine. Speak to your healthcare practitioner to help ascertain the risk. Normally, vaccination at a hospital with resuscitation equipment at close hand can be arranged.

Holidays and travel

With all the anxiety of living with food allergy, you probably deserve a break more than most. Advance thinking is essential when it comes to getting away from it all. Don't leave matters until the last minute. Plan for all eventualities.

Before you go

Choose destinations sympathetic to your allergies. If you're dairy- or wheat-allergic, south-east Asia may be suitable, whereas Italy, land of pasta, pizza and Parmesan, may not. If you're soya-allergic, the reverse applies. Bear in mind that non-developed countries are likely to have exceptionally low allergy rates, and your condition may not always be appreciated.

Touristy areas, such as Spanish resorts, are likely to be populated with more English speakers – helpful if you're nervous about the language barrier. Ask your travel agent about hotels catering for those on restricted diets. If you have multiple or severe allergies, self-catering may be the better option. An hour or more spent online researching your chosen location – its dishes, restaurants, health food stores, hotels – will be well worthwhile.

Acquire translations to common culprits. *Foods Matter* magazine supplies food list translations in several European languages, and Allergy UK offers laminated alert cards in around 30 languages to show restaurant staff. If you're travelling to a country whose main tongue is not covered by these services, consider having some phrases such as 'I am severely allergic to . . .' or 'Is this product guaranteed free from . . . ?' translated through a reputable translation agency (find one in the Yellow Pages). If you have any other idiosyncratic medical requirements that may need to be communicated to healthcare workers while abroad, ask your doctor to write a succinct summary, which again you could have translated. You may want to do likewise with your emergency action plan, copies of which you can later give to hotel management and your tour reps or guides.

Pack essential safe supplies such as allergen-free snacks in case you're caught short, say by flight delays, and take cosmetic items such as sun lotion too. The less shopping you have to do in a foreign country, the better. Within EU countries, you may be able to make sense of ingredients with the help of your translations or a phrasebook, but elsewhere labelling can be anarchic. Foreign versions of foods found on UK shelves may contain varying ingredients and will be made in a different factory, even if the brand is identical, so a safe product at home may not be a safe product away.

Ensure you have enough adrenaline (and other medication); obtaining replacements abroad could be laborious. Check with your travel agent and airline that injectors are allowed in the cabin, and arrange a verifying letter from your doctor to produce at security control or check-in. Remember to pack storage cases for your medication: adrenaline can degrade in the heat of the beach, so you need to protect it carefully.

Ensure your travel insurance covers treatment for your allergy, and obtain a European Health Insurance Card (www.ehic.org.uk; 0845 606 2030), which has replaced the old E111 form, before you travel within the EU. Wearing conspicuous MedicAlert jewellery gives foreign doctors the opportunity to call a number to access your medical details through an interpreter in an emergency.

Air travel

An aeroplane mid-flight is one of the last places you would choose to experience a reaction, and many people liable to have severe allergic reactions are, understandably, worried about flying.

Speak to your travel agent or, much better, call and deal with the airline directly. Some airlines operate nut-free catering policies, and some – like BA and Aer Lingus – do not serve peanuts, but they cannot stop other passengers bringing snacks on board. Airborne nut allergens can trigger reactions, but only mild ones usually. Snacks handed out with drinks are more of a concern, as this will cause greater volumes of allergens to circulate in the cabin atmosphere. Nevertheless, the risk remains low. It's worth taking along some wet wipes to clean seats and fold-down trays in the event of nut traces left behind from an earlier flight.

The most likely cause of a reaction is through consumption. The best security is to bring your own food.

When you come to fly, let check-in staff and senior members of cabin crew know of your allergy. The more people you inform, the more likely your needs will be accommodated.

When you arrive

As soon as is convenient, speak to your rep, hotel manager and anyone else involved in your care during your holiday. Give them as much information about your condition as possible. Discuss the best action in an emergency in different situations – when you're at the beach, on a day trip, at the hotel. Learn the correct ambulance emergency number, such as 911 in America and Canada, and 112 in much of Europe.

Ask about health shops or natural food stores locally – either at the hotel or at tourist information – as you will need to stock up on safe foods. Assistants here are also likely to be more knowledgeable about restricted diets than those in supermarkets, and your translations will be handy. Visit them soon so you get to know them, or can find alternative stockists if they're unsuitable.

Don't put these errands off – the sooner you get them done and reassure yourself, the longer you can devote to relaxation.

Eating abroad

One of the toughest aspects of holidaying abroad is having to navigate the culinary wonders that mercilessly tempt your senses – markets and bazaars heady with the intoxicating aromas of street food, for instance, and delicatessen windows displaying magical ethnic delights.

The level of care you take depends largely on the severity of your condition. If you do wish to taste local foods or dishes, ask as many questions as you need to, use your translation cards and ensure you have your medication to hand. When eating out, it may be worth dining outside peak lunch or dinner hours, when waiters and chefs will be less harassed and more able to cater for you precisely.

Take care not only with prepared foods, but also unfamiliar raw fruits and vegetables. African, South American and Caribbean countries, in particular, boast a lot of native produce which never reaches these shores, but which may cross-react with your particular allergens. If you have latex–fruit cross-reactions, bear in mind that other tropical fruits, besides those which you know trigger a response, may also be reactive.

Lots of nations or cultures have their own idiosyncratic food traditions, products and delicacies, and it is impossible to list all potential dangers. For instance, almonds and almond flour are liberally used in Spain, Portugal and some Latin American countries in pastries, cakes and other baked goods. Lupin flour is used widely in France, the Mediterranean and Australia, and in Greece, the beans and seeds are consumed as foods and snacks in their own right. Wheat beers, as well as the usual barley-based beers, are common in Germany and in the Benelux countries – watch out for the terms Hefeweizen, Weissbier or Kristallweizen in German-speaking nations.

As always, you just have to be on your guard.

6
Coping emotionally

The psychological effects of food allergy are little discussed, and yet the impact on those affected and those nearest to them can be huge – something clinicians are only now appreciating. When so much of your life is spent on the practical implications of your condition – carrying medication, monitoring labels – it's easy, but ultimately unwise, to neglect your emotional health.

Coping with diagnosis

Why me? Is it something I did wrong? These are often the first thoughts of sufferers when they receive confirmation of what they've perhaps suspected for a while. Be assured that in no way are you to blame for your allergy. You, or your child, just got unlucky.

You may feel shocked at this 'failure' of your body, and unable to take in the implications of what you've learned, or you may feel vindicated in discovering that your reactions haven't been 'all in the mind'. In those who have been seeking a diagnosis for many months, that relief may be short-lived – the stress of not knowing what was wrong and perhaps trying to convince your doctor that something was amiss may have been lifted, but now it has been replaced with the anxiety of an uncertain future.

Obviously the most desirable response to diagnosis is a positive, combative one, where you decide to arm yourself with knowledge and tackle the illness head on, refusing to let it get the better of you. It's also beneficial to assess your support network and 'rally the troops' – your personal retinue of partner, friends and family, who care for you and can help you come to terms with your condition.

That said, some people, through no fault of their own, find the road to this stage a bumpy one.

Self-pity

A brief period spent feeling sorry for yourself can do you good: if you're overwhelmed with your diagnosis and its implications, having a short 'shut down' for a few days could be just what you need, and is perfectly normal. Allow yourself time off work. When you emerge from the gloom, as you begin to accept your situation, you will probably find yourself ready to do battle with your allergy.

Shock and anger

You may feel resentful of the situation in which you find yourself, and may take your frustration out on loved ones. These feelings are normal, and will usually pass quickly.

Denial and indifference

Consider these attitudes:

- 'It's only a bit of tingling and wheezing – I'll be OK so long as I don't eat nuts at the pub any more.'
- 'There's no cure and nothing I can do about it. I'll just put up with the reactions and carry on as normal. I don't really care.'
- 'I'll be fine. My family and friends will watch out for me.'

Denying a problem, adopting a recklessly carefree stance, passing the onus of responsibility on to loved ones – these are all common initial responses, especially in teenagers.

While they might act as 'stepping stones' to help temporarily defuse the shock of the initial blow of diagnosis, beware the danger of prolonged denial. If you've read this far, it's unlikely you have such an issue, but these attitudes are worth looking out for if you're a parent of youngsters. Parents and medical professionals must ensure, sympathetically but firmly, that young allergic patients are clear on what they can and can't eat, what the risks are, and so on.

Ongoing emotional problems

Some people, especially those with mild or non-life-threatening conditions, take food allergy completely in their stride. Others experience occasional or chronic psychological problems or hardships, and it is important be aware of these possibilities.

Complacency

This is a sign that denial is creeping back.
Ask yourself these questions:

- Have you taken to regularly ignoring food labels?
- Are you beginning to take risks with products carrying 'may contain' warnings?
- Do you often catch yourself thinking, 'Just this once won't hurt'?
- Have you allowed yourself to slip into a 'take it or leave it' attitude towards your medication?
- Do you increasingly avoid telling people about your condition?
- Have you stopped visiting your doctor to discuss your allergy?

The more 'yes' responses, the more likely you are to be sliding into perilous territory. A reaction can often act as a wake-up call in such circumstances, but it is preferable to identify lapses and nip them in the bud.

Although it can affect everyone, teenagers, especially boys, are more susceptible. Seeing themselves as young and immortal, having possibly avoided serious reactions for many years thanks to the vigilance of their parents, and wanting to live a normal lifestyle, they are more likely to expose themselves to high-risk situations. Sadly, some individuals keep their risk-taking from friends and family, both to protect them from worry and, ironically, to avoid giving others the idea that their allergy is less serious than it actually is.

Shame and stigma

Tragically, many sufferers feel deeply embarrassed, even stigmatized, by their condition – some report feeling like 'freaks' among their non-allergic acquaintances. The distorted perception and widespread ignorance of food allergy among the population compounds the problem. People may be sceptical, unsympathetic, and may make you feel conspicuously 'different'. Having to speak to chefs before dining, or standing up to colleagues who are pressuring you to join them for a Thai meal, is tough.

Sufferers can react to this in two ways: avoiding social situations and isolating themselves; or 'going with the flow', ignoring their illness and taking risks. Both are causes for concern.

Depression

Not all people perceive depression as an illness: for some, it's a choice made on the back of finding oneself in tough circumstances. Indeed, a period of mild depressive withdrawal can act protectively. But when this stretches indefinitely, the situation becomes serious.

Those at particular risk include those in middle-to-late age, for whom living with a food allergy can have resonant symbolic overtones. If you're older, allergic illness may make you feel doubly fragile at a time when your body might already be showing other signs of failing. This vulnerability can be much more debilitating than the practical implications of suddenly having to avoid a food.

Symptoms of depression include:

- indifference, including to pleasurable activities;
- lethargy and tiredness;
- disordered sleep and rest patterns;
- reduced appetite or, conversely, comfort eating;
- low concentration and motivation;
- overwhelming feelings of inadequacy, uselessness, hopelessness;
- loss of self-confidence;
- sadness;
- irritability and restlessness.

Anxiety and stress

These are common and often severe.

Some anxiety is important: from an evolutionary perspective, stress is a survivalist trait to keep you alert to possible danger and primed to respond to it. For instance, it is vital you maintain a low, constant level of vigilance to avoid allergens, and be able to promptly respond to an accidental exposure. Don't look upon stress as all bad.

That said, chronic stress can be debilitating, and is a sign of a problem which needs resolving. Parents of food-allergic children are known to suffer extreme, relentless anxiety, and the pressure of living under what is perceived to be a constant threat can be too much for food-allergic adults too. Stress also compounds asthma and eczema symptoms.

Symptoms of anxiety include:

- a dry mouth;
- cold or hot sweats;

- changes in eating habits;
- inability to work or concentrate;
- sleep disturbance;
- sexual disinterest or dysfunction;
- obviously untrue negative thoughts.

Fear

A natural response. Allergy sufferers may fear all manner of things – being surprised by an unexpected kiss from a fish-loving friend, having to self-inject adrenaline, or dying of a severe reaction. Fear can be justified, or it can be disproportionate to the actual threat, but the feelings can be equally intense either way.

Panic

Adult food allergy sufferers may be more at risk of suffering from panic attacks, possibly triggered by something such as the sudden realization during a night out at a restaurant that they have forgotten their medication. The symptoms – chest tightness, fighting for air, hyperventilation, dizziness, visual disturbances – can be sudden and acutely distressing. Sufferers often feel as if they are about to die, which can further perpetuate symptoms.

Eating disorders

Little research has been done looking at a link between eating disorders and food allergy, but anecdotal evidence appears to show there is one. Studies suggest that those self-diagnosing their allergies demonstrate higher than average levels of anorexia nervosa and bulimia, though it is unclear whether the eating disorders follow on from the 'allergy', or whether claims of allergy are adopted by some women to legitimize their food exclusions. Media coverage of svelte personalities who have supposedly overcome sensitivities may be partly to blame.

It is also possible that the great care that some genuine food-allergics need to take with their diets may, in vulnerable individuals, gradually slip towards hyper-obsessiveness, extreme food exclusions and, consequently, anorexic-type behaviour.

Becoming obsessed with your diet or size, being disturbed by minor weight gain, depression, social withdrawal, and excessive exercise are all signs of a problem.

Food aversion

This is a psychological adverse reaction towards food, occurring when the sufferer becomes mistakenly convinced that one or more foods cause food allergy symptoms. Because they may go on to needlessly eliminate supposed allergens from their diet, some people then run the risk of malnutrition or eating disorders. An incidence of food poisoning or a mistaken diagnosis from a fringe practitioner can act as the 'trigger' to an aversion.

Obsessive Compulsive Disorder (OCD)

Although allergic children are less likely than adults to suffer from stress and anxiety, they are more susceptible to OCD. It may be that the hypervigilance demanded by their illness spills into other areas of their lives, promoting wider obsessive behaviour.

Trauma

If you have lived through the ordeal of a severe anaphylactic reaction you may feel devastated by the experience. The shock of the 'near miss', of perhaps coming close to death, can undermine your stability and be emotionally disabling. People who've ticked along for years with perhaps only minor reactions or none at all can feel especially traumatized if an anaphylactic episode has hit them like a bolt from the blue.

Post-traumatic stress disorder (PTSD) is unlikely in those who have suffered anaphylactic reactions, but not impossible. Flashbacks or powerful visualizations – such as of your ambulance dash, or emergency treatment – being unable to follow simple, day-to-day routine, hypervigilance and obsessiveness, disrupted sleep and nightmares, and violent behaviour – can all be symptoms.

Self-help

Although there are plenty of individuals, specialists and groups who can help, you are undoubtedly the most important person involved in your own emotional care.

Knowledge and positivity

Learn about your allergy, and approach your fact-finding mission positively; your aim is to eliminate the anxiety ignorance breeds.

Remind yourself too that your condition, despite perhaps being serious, is absolutely manageable.

Statistics can offer great reassurance: for instance, over a million people in this country are avoiding nuts, almost a quarter of a million carry adrenaline, and yet there are only on average about eight deaths annually from anaphylaxis, tragic though these are. Relatively speaking, your risks are low.

If there is something you do not understand, a niggling query which is bothering you, then resolve to find the answer – if this book can't help, ask your healthcare professional, or call an allergy charity.

Also, try to learn from reactions you have, and see the positive aspects of them. Some people who endure an anaphylactic reaction and successfully rescue themselves with an EpiPen come to feel empowered by the experience, and reassured in the knowledge that they can manage even the worst of incidents.

Positive thinking also helps your self-esteem and self-confidence, which may be dented by your allergic status. Be proud, not ashamed, when you need to tell, say, waiting staff of your illness, and don't be afraid to put it in no-nonsense terms that you have a life-threatening condition. Practise in front of a mirror. Or consider taking assertiveness classes if you feel this is a problem area.

Volunteering

Helping yourself by helping others can work wonders. Volunteering 'gives something back' to the allergic community, and will also strengthen your character and prove deeply fulfilling.

Allergy UK, for instance, runs a 'support contact' scheme, where volunteers undertake to act as a point of contact for local people living with allergies, to keep in regular touch and swap tips and information. The charity also encourages and supports members to organize fundraising events, or you could perhaps consider other options, such as giving a talk at your local school to kids and teachers about food allergy, which may also be rewarding.

Writing therapy

Putting your thoughts, anxieties and fears down on paper is an excellent way of clearing your head, unburdening yourself, under-standing your problems and charting your emotional progress.

Consider finding an allergic penfriend, keeping a diary or even starting a 'blog' – an online web diary of your experiences of food allergy, which may well attract attention from other sufferers worldwide.

Relaxation and breathing

Many people complain of being unable to relax, but there is more to unwinding than merely willing yourself to do so. Pampering – a hot bath, aromatherapy oils – can help, as can a massage from a willing partner. Meditation, prayer and chanting are deeply relaxing; as are forms of yoga and healing martial arts such as t'ai chi. Find what works for you, and remember that relaxation takes practice.

For instant stress-relief if you're feeling uptight or nervous, try a technique of 'expanding' your peripheral vision. Find a point opposite you, just above eye-level, and keeping your eyes on that point, begin to slowly broaden your field of vision to notice more of what's on either side of the point, so that eventually you're paying attention to that which is visible in the corners of your eyes. You should begin to feel your breathing moving lower in your chest, slowing down, becoming deeper, and your facial muscles relaxing. Very calming.

Indeed, learning to breathe correctly is of enormous value to stress-relief: inhale deeply and slowly into the belly to the count of three, exhale evenly to the count of three, then pause for one – and repeat. Yogic breathing while seated and focusing on a lighted candle is very soothing.

If you suffer panic attacks, focusing on good breathing practice can reduce the symptoms caused by hyperventilation during acutely stressful moments.

Friends and family

The role of loved ones in your psychological care should never be underestimated.

Good friends ...

You need around you positive people who can offer practical advice and emotional support, who can lift your gloom and bring laughter into your life when you feel there is none, and who make you feel understood. The most valuable are the people who know your needs, the implications of your illness, can act as your personal 'body-guards' should your own guard slip – and who don't make any demands in return. According to relationships expert and motivational speaker Paul McGee, creator of the SUMO (Shut Up, Move On) principles for personal development, the best friends to have are 'radiators' – reliable, there when you need them, able to provide you with warmth.

But that doesn't mean all your friends should be Mary Poppins clones. You also need people who are unafraid to give you difficult truths when they apply – to point out that you are foolishly taking risks with certain foods, or that you may benefit from seeking professional help with your mental health, for instance.

Shutting people out is a never-win situation. Most who care for you will want to help in any way they can, so don't be too proud to ask for practical help or a shoulder to cry on. You may feel you want to protect family members from the burden of your illness, but, again, most prefer to be involved – even if it's just by giving you a ride to the allergy clinic.

... and not so good friends

Understand that not everyone you meet, work with or are friendly with will be helpful or supportive, often through ignorance not malice. Some people will not get the allergy 'scene', and will insist that 'allergies are all in the mind' because an article they once read said so. Upsetting as this may be, it will probably always be the way to some extent, and arguing the case may not always prove fruitful, or make you feel better.

All friends have their strengths and weaknesses, and a much valued confidant may not necessarily be the right one to turn to when you're suffering problems related to your allergy. Paul McGee warns against three types to avoid when the going gets tough:

- 'The Happy' – who trivializes your allergy and tells you not to be silly, that it's nothing to worry about;
- 'The Hijacker' – who takes over and tells you about his problems with ill health when you ask for support with yours;
- 'The Awfulizer' – who is alarmed at your condition and treats it like a crippling handicap or threatening death sentence.

Be aware of these, and of other people who make you feel worse – such as those who appear to enjoy the 'fuss' of your illness, or who seem to be bored by or indifferent towards it.

Support groups

Occasionally, you may feel more comfortable seeking the support of strangers rather than that of loved ones.

Charities

The allergy charities have superb helplines manned by supportive, knowledgeable people who can offer emotional as well as practical support.

Other groups from whose services you may benefit include:

- The National Phobics Society (0870 122 2325; www.phobics-society.org.uk) – for anxiety disorders and phobias;
- NoPanic (0808 808 0545; www.nopanic.org.uk) – for panic attacks, phobias, OCD and anxiety disorders;
- Assist (01788 560800; www.traumatic-stress.freeserve.co.uk) – for victims of trauma;
- Stress Anxiety Depression Helpline (01622 717656) – for self-help strategies, therapies and guidance for stress disorders;
- The Eating Disorders Association (0845 634 1414; www.edauk. com) – for anorexia, bulimia and other eating disorders;
- SupportLine (020 8554 9004; www.supportline.org.uk) – for confidential emotional support, and details of other agencies, groups and counsellors in the country.

Meetings, activities and workshops

Taking part in social or learning events designed for people living with allergies is an ideal opportunity to relieve the isolation you may be feeling, meet people in the same boat as you – because there are many – and lift your spirits.

The Anaphylaxis Campaign is especially active in this area, helping to organize local support-group meetings throughout the country, as well as workshops and breaks for parents and teenagers, and activity holidays for children – especially valuable in helping youngsters overcome some of the psychological obstacles typical of their age group, such as embarrassment or OCD, and indeed boost their confidence levels.

Online support groups

The internet revolution has seen a number of groups dedicated to people with food allergies spring up online – see 'Useful addresses'.

People who live in secluded areas and feel isolated, those who are disabled, or single parents of young children, are among those who find these groups of particular value – but they can help anyone who perhaps is shy or has difficulty with face-to-face contact, and prefers the anonymity the web and e-mail can offer.

Although groups can be extremely encouraging and supportive, be sure to choose one with a knowledgeable moderator, who will remove any suspect, offensive or dangerous postings.

Professional help

Sometimes, stubborn psychological problems need to be referred a step further.

Your doctor

Doctors are your first port of call if you're suffering symptoms of stress, depression, anxiety, or are concerned with other areas of your psychological health. They are trained to see signs of emotional difficulties in their patients, and ideally placed to advise on possible private treatments or referrals. Do make use of your GP; many have good counselling skills and unburdening yourself to them may be all you need.

Your dietitian

If you're anxious about food avoidance or nutrition, a dietitian can help fill the gaps in your knowledge and offer excellent guidance and reassurance.

Dietitians may also have a role to play in identifying and helping resolve possible eating disorders and aversions.

Your allergy consultant

Your most complex queries can almost certainly be answered by your allergy consultant, with whom you should try to develop an active relationship. The more knowledge you demonstrate, and the more questions you ask of specialists, the more likely you will be given greater detail and reassurance. If you feel burdened by not knowing whether or not you are still allergic to a particular food, a consultant can arrange further testing.

'Talking' therapists

If your doctor feels you need more specialized help, referral for counselling or psychotherapy may be suggested. There are few specialists working in these fields in the NHS, so a private referral may be required.

There are few differences between the talking therapies, even though counselling sounds – and is – gentler and less demanding than psychotherapy. Both involve face-to-face meetings with a trained therapist to reach any number of end goals, depending entirely on the patient, such as the reduction of psychological distress and the promotion of emotional health.

Counsellors will listen to you, aim to identify with you and your dilemmas, help you clarify them in your mind, and perhaps give advice – although generally their aim is to help you to discover your own answers to your problems through carefully guided discussion. Counsellors can, for instance, help patients cope and come to terms with difficult events like diagnosis.

Psychotherapists, of whom there are many kinds, work similarly, but use more analytical approaches and explore difficulties in greater depth. They may work with those suffering from depression, anxiety and addictive behaviour disorders, those who are finding it difficult to adjust to allergic illness, those whose condition is impacting on many areas of their life, or anyone traumatized by an anaphylactic experience.

These therapies are presently unregulated in the UK, and so look for accreditation in your therapist if you are taking the solo route privately. Membership of the British Association for Counselling and Psychotherapy (BACP – 0870 443 5252; www.bacp.co.uk), the UK Council for Psychotherapy (UKCP – 020 7014 9955; www. psychotherapy.org.uk), or the United Kingdom Register of Counsellors (UKRC – www.ukrconline.org.uk) is important.

Make sure you have an assessment session, and discontinue any therapy with a specialist with whom you feel uncomfortable – being at ease with your counsellor is vital. Remember too that counselling is not easy, or a magic wand: expect positive changes but not miracles. Some people approach therapy expecting their stresses to be entirely removed, but therapists will not do this: they will arm you with coping mechanisms, not seek to abolish all your responses.

Cognitive behaviour therapy (CBT)

CBT is an objective psychotherapeutic approach which is less interested in what caused your emotional or psychological difficulties, and more concerned with how you handle your dilemmas. It challenges the negative thought patterns which may be causing your problems, helps you identify and understand them, equips you with coping skills, and implements changes to unhelpful thinking or behaviour. The therapy is structured, practical and result-focused, unlike counselling which usually involves 'freer' conversation and a greater rapport with the therapist.

CBT might be right for those looking for help with a specific issue. It is useful for depression, phobias or stress, for example, where the emphasis may be on cognition or thinking; while for eating disorders or OCD, predominantly behavioural issues will be tackled.

The British Association of Behavioural and Cognitive Psychotherapies (BABCP – 01254 875277; www.babcp.com) has a register of qualified CBT practitioners.

Hypnotherapy

This is a psychotherapy which uses hypnosis – a state of deep relaxation and heightened awareness, which makes the mind more receptive to positive suggestion. It can help those suffering from low self-esteem, phobias, panic, anxiety and OCD, for example. You are unlikely to get hypnotherapy on the NHS, but it is usually considerably cheaper than, say, CBT. Always look out for accredited individuals. The National Register of Hypnotherapists and Psychotherapists (NRHP – 01282 716839; www.nrhp.co.uk) and the National Council for Hypnotherapy (0800 952 0545; www.hypnotherapists.org.uk) can help.

7

Nutrition and health

You may be worried about the effects reactions and dietary limitations have on your health. Rest assured that no matter how many food restrictions you have or how serious your symptoms, there is plenty you can do to keep yourself in optimal mental and physical shape.

Allergen-free nutrition

Living with food allergy generally means living on a restricted diet, and living on a restricted diet may compromise your nutrition. Usually, though, introducing wholesome replacement foods into your eating plans and making other modest changes will ensure you don't suffer any deficiencies.

Tree nuts, peanuts and seeds

It's a bitter irony that these often dangerously allergic foods happen to be among the most nutritious. Nuts and seeds are rich in proteins and essential fatty acids (EFAs), B vitamins, vitamin E, calcium and many important trace minerals which are sometimes lacking in Western diets.

Even if you are avoiding all varieties, however, there are unlikely to be any serious negative consequences on your health. Seafood, especially oily fish, offers a source of valuable EFAs, and you could look at including *refined* seed oils – which should be free of allergenic proteins – into your diet.

Other sources of trace minerals include barley, liver and seafood (for copper), brown rice, wholemeal bread, fish and chicken (selenium), and meat, dairy, eggs, fish and soya (zinc). Avocados are a good source of vitamin E, a natural anti-inflammatory and powerful antioxidant which may help mildly dampen reactions.

Fish and seafood

These are rich in protein, minerals such as iodine and – especially in the case of oily fish – omega-3 fatty acids, celebrated for their many beneficial effects, including cardiovascular functioning and psychological and mental well-being.

If you must omit seafood, incorporate olives, nuts and seeds such as flax, hemp, rape and walnuts – or their oils – into your diet. Liver and offal are also rich in omega 3s, as are some new 'functional' foods, such as omega 3-rich eggs. Products *fortified* with fish oils, such as some cereal bars, breads, milks and juices, or indeed fish oil supplements, are potential triggers for very severely fish-allergic people, and should be avoided.

Dairy produce

Calcium intake is the main concern if you're allergic to dairy foods. Most soya milks are calcium-enriched, but sardines and other bony fish, tofu, green vegetables (broccoli, spinach) and nuts are good alternative sources. Adequate vitamin D (from eggs, oily fish and sunlight) helps calcium's uptake by the body.

Yoghurt provides probiotic bacteria, which may help to maintain intestinal health. In its absence, you may like to consider other sources, such as sauerkraut and soya miso. French company Sojasun produce soya-based probiotic drinks, available from Goodness Direct.

Prebiotics – carbohydrates on which probiotics feed – can encourage the growth and reproduction of health-giving intestinal flora. Sources are bananas, members of the lily family (onion, garlic, asparagus), and some members of the daisy family (chicory, Jerusalem artichokes).

Wheat

Despite its poor reputation among alternative therapists, wheat is a source of protein, starchy carbohydrates, fibre, B vitamins and minerals – and therefore an excellent all-round food. All its nutrients are vital to the body's many biological processes, but can be obtained from a varied diet of meat, dairy foods, eggs, nuts, pulses and seeds, fruit and vegetables – and other cereals.

Try unrefined whole-grains such as brown rice, and experiment with nutritious grains such as amaranth, millet and quinoa, which rarely trigger allergies. Starchy vegetables such as potato, sweet potato and other tubers, and corn and polenta (Italian maize meal), constitute good carbohydrate replacements too.

Eggs

Eggs contain vitamins A and B, protein and some zinc, but having to eliminate them from your diet is unlikely to leave you deficient in a nutrient obtainable from an otherwise broad diet including meat, dairy or legumes.

Soya

A good vegetarian source of protein, and a useful source of calcium and other minerals. Although tough to avoid, omitting soya should not be problematic nutritionally: other legumes – such as peas and lentils – can compensate.

Fruit and vegetables

These provide vitamins (especially vitamin C, a natural antihist-amine), fibre (both soluble and insoluble) and some trace minerals. Dark or brightly coloured fruits and vegetables are also rich in antioxidant chemicals, understood to boost immunity and protect against a wide range of illnesses – everything from colds to forms of cancer.

It's important to eat a selection of safe fruit and vegetables when you're excluding others, especially because research suggests that many people with allergy have reduced antioxidant status. One particular antioxidant of interest in allergy is quercetin, reputed to have a calming, anti-inflammatory effect; it is found in onions, cranberries, apples and red grapes.

Most fruit-allergic people experience mild reactions to multiple fruits which are related to pollen sensitivity, and can eat tinned or cooked fruit, pasteurized juices and sometimes peeled fruits. Raw fruits rarely implicated in cross-reactions with pollens and which are therefore usually safe include grapes, pomegranates, figs, many currants and berries, and citrus fruits.

Latex-allergic people with associated allergies to tropical fruits are more likely to find native and European fruits such as apples, pears, berries, grapes and citrus fruits tolerable.

Those experiencing reactions to fruits unrelated to either pollen or latex sensitivity are less likely to be multiply sensitive and so will have more choice in alternatives.

Nutritional deficiencies are improbable if a broad range of vegetables (cooked if necessary) are also consumed.

Responses to vegetables are rare and generally resolved by cooking when pollen sensitivity is the cause, celery being an occasional exception. Having to avoid a particular type will not have nutritional consequences provided you eat many others. However, those with tomato allergy may be missing out on the red antioxidant lycopene, which has purported anti-cancer potential. Other, more moderate, sources which you could include if you don't react to them are watermelon, pink grapefruit and guava.

Eating a healthy diet

So much is written nowadays about eating healthily that the consumer can easily become overwhelmed with the unnecessarily detailed and sometimes contradictory advice given. It's easy to form the impression that sound nutrition is complex. It isn't. In reality, sticking to a few basic principles should ensure you maintain good dietary habits.

Possibly the most important is variety: try to eat as diverse a diet as possible within the parameters of your exclusions. Avoid coming to rely on any one 'safe' food which provides only a limited range of nutrients; over-consumption can also increase your risk of becoming intolerant to a food.

How you eat is vital too. Take your time – when you're selecting food, cooking it and most importantly eating it. Eat when you're calm and relaxed and can focus on your meal, not when you're rushed or anxious or distracted, when mistakes and oversights are more likely. Remain quietly vigilant and on guard – always. Take care not to become complacent about eating habits – continue to check ingredients and monitor your diet.

Also, don't skip meals, especially breakfast – you'll experience uncomfortable fluctuations in energy and blood sugar levels, and you'll be more vulnerable to casual snacking and grabbing possibly unsafe convenience foods on the go. Plan ahead, and always have healthy and safe foods to hand should you be caught short and peckish.

And remember: just because you have a food allergy doesn't mean you can't be passionate about food. Learn to cook new dishes. Interest yourself in food news and culinary innovations. Live to eat; don't eat to live.

Essential foods

Several food groups are key to your diet.

Complex carbohydrates

These include all grains, and the foods based on them, such as pastas, breads and cereal products. Potatoes also fall into this category. Roughly eight to ten daily servings are recommended to ensure adequate intake of slow energy-releasing carbohydrates and of fibre. A slice of bread, an egg-sized potato, three tablespoons of cereal and two heaped tablespoons of rice count as a serving each.

Protein foods

Two to three servings of either meat, fish, eggs, beans, nuts or seeds are advised. A portion is equivalent to 100g of meat or fish, two eggs, three tablespoons of beans or a handful of nuts and seeds.

Fruit and vegetables

As these are essential sources of carbohydrates, fibre, vitamins, minerals and antioxidant chemicals, you should aim to consume at least five portions daily, preferably more. A handful of berries, an apple, a banana, three tablespoons of peas or lentils, and a side salad are each roughly equivalent to one portion.

Dairy foods

While not strictly essential, two or three servings of either milk, yoghurt or cheese are recommended by dietitians – provided of course you don't have a dairy allergy. A matchbox-sized chunk of cheese, a small pot of yoghurt or a small glass of milk each provide a serving.

Water

Two litres daily is the often-quoted figure to which we should supposedly all aspire, but the quantity depends on so many different factors – the size of the individual, the amount of activity undertaken, the temperature and environment – that it's misleading to generalize.

A good barometer of healthy and adequate hydration is the colour of your urine. Too dark signifies you may lack fluids, so aim to drink enough to keep your pee straw-coloured. Water itself is the best hydrator, but fruit juices, squashes, sodas and milk all contain mostly water and count towards your quota. As do, within reason, teas, coffees and colas – the dehydrating effects of the caffeine in these drinks being absurdly exaggerated by many complementary therapists but negligible in reality. Alcoholic drinks, which dehydrate heavily, certainly do not count.

Non-essential foods

In moderation, other foods have their place in the context of a healthy diet, but take care not to overindulge.

Caffeine

Moderate caffeine consumption is safe for most people, and perhaps even beneficial to asthmatics, but avoid drinking more than three to four cups of coffee daily in order to stay within recommended guidelines, and remember that black and green teas, cola, cocoa and chocolate products, as well as some painkillers, contain caffeine.

Sugar

Cakes, biscuits, pastries, chocolate bars, sweets – most of us love occasional treats, and they're important for your psychological health, especially if you're feeling down about dietary limitations. Eat sugar sparingly, though – no more than 10 per cent of your daily calories should come from sugar, which is roughly equivalent to 50g or twelve level teaspoons. Read labels carefully for added sugars.

Alcohol

Moderate alcohol consumption – up to three units a day – is generally considered OK. The universal health risks of excessive alcohol consumption aside, as a food-allergic you need to take extra care as drinking can reduce your vigilance and dull your senses and responses, leaving you more liable to let your guard slip, thoughtlessly consume a reactive food, and also delay in recognizing and treating symptoms.

Convenience food and 'bad' fats

Although fat intake has no obvious direct relevance to food-allergic people, for other health reasons it's wise to limit your intake of junk foods and saturated fats, typically found in rich cuts of meat, dairy products such as butter and cream, and any number of desserts and sweet products.

Trans fats are a particular class of fats manufactured during hydrogenation – a process which converts liquid vegetable oils into solid fats and margarines. Many researchers consider them unhealthier than saturated fats. Typically, trans fats are found in pastries, cakes, biscuits, convenience meat products such as pies, and takeaway foods. Some manufacturers have now removed trans fats from their margarines.

Of course, some fats are needed in the diet, and unsaturated fats – found in fish, nuts, seeds, avocados and vegetable oils such as olive oils – are best.

'Free-from' foods

These have their place, and can be very useful, but they may contain high levels of refined carbohydrates, fats and additives. Wheat-free products especially are worth scrutinizing. Use modestly, and ask yourself whether the product is a good food in its own right. Would you eat it if you weren't suffering from food allergy?

Organic food

There is some evidence that organic food is healthier than non-organic, but the advantage may be marginal. In those with oral allergies to fruit and vegetables, symptoms when eating organic versions may be milder because it's possible that pesticides used on non-organic produce cause plants to manufacture greater quantities of 'defensive' allergens.

Supplementation

In certain circumstances, nutritional supplements may be suggested or advised – but take your cue from your doctor or dietitian. Avoid supplementing without specialist advice, never assume you can compensate for omitted foods with vitamin pills, and don't use supplements as substitutes for skipped meals. Always verify supplements are allergen-free.

Do I need to see a dietitian?

Dietitians can advise on allergen avoidance, and on ensuring you follow a nutritionally adequate diet. Some have a special interest in food allergy.

On the NHS you need a referral from your doctor to see one, and waiting lists can be long. A consultation should be granted if you have multiple allergies or additional dietary restrictions due to medical, ethical or religious reasons, when following a healthy diet could be tricky. If, for example, you're a vegan with allergies to nuts, seeds and legumes, it's likely you'll need specialist advice on ensuring sufficient protein intake.

In most cases involving children, especially those with dairy allergy, seeing a dietitian for advice is important.

You can elect to see one privately if you are concerned about your nutrition: to find one, see www.dietitiansunlimited. co.uk, or contact the allergy charities. Ensure your dietitian is state registered and be wary of fringe therapists also calling themselves nutritionists. The Health Professions Council hold a database of state-registered dietitians at www.hpc.uk.org or call them on 020 7582 0866.

Health and your immune system

Given that in allergy your immune system is inappropriately sensitive to certain proteins, looking after it may, some propose, reduce the severity of your responses and help you recover from reactions more quickly. Although the reasoning of this argument may be sound, there's little evidence to suggest the effect is marked in practice. All the same, taking care of your overall health and immune system is certainly worthwhile. Other than eating healthily, here are some additional tips.

- Take regular exercise. Ensure it's something you enjoy, not find a chore. If the gym doesn't do it for you, find something which does. Just 30 minutes vigorous activity, three times a week, can help cardiovascular health.

- Ditch the cigarettes and cigars – for too many reasons to mention, not forgetting their effect on the immune system. See www. givingupsmoking.co.uk.
- Don't work excessively. We have a five-day, 35-hour week for a reason. Burning the midnight oil makes it impossible for you to savour much-needed down-time. Switch off your computer and your mobile, and go for a relaxing stroll or play with the kids instead.
- Keep stress levels low. Anxiety suppresses immunity. Yoga, meditation, massage, a soothing bath, sex – all help you to wind down, especially at the end of a working day.
- Get your eight hours of shut-eye. Sleep deprivation can make you feel run down and lower your immune defences. Those living with allergies need to keep as alert as possible. If you don't get a full night's kip, take ten-minute catnaps during the day.
- Show emotion and express your feelings: bottling it all up is psychologically and physiologically damaging.
- Breathe clean air. Minimize exposure to pollutants and chemical substances, both inside and outside the home. For instance, avoid jogging in rush hour or near main roads, and try using natural cleansers in the home, such as lemon juice.
- Keep a low-allergen home. Vacuum at least once a week to clear dust, mites and pet dander; wash curtains, as they can trap pollen; check all corners of humid rooms for any mould; change and launder bedding and sheets regularly to keep bed bugs and their allergenic droppings to a minimum.
- And finally ... laugh – and laugh some more. Watch back-to-back episodes of favourite comedies or spend weekends with entertaining friends. Laughter is not the best medicine, but it is certainly a very good one – and scientific research is supporting this view.

8

Treatments and prevention

If only we could make all allergies go away when they materialized, or, even better, stop them developing in the first place, then this book might not be needed. Unfortunately, such medical progress could be some time off yet.

Treatments

The science of treating food allergic individuals with a view to reducing their future responses to triggers or curing them of their allergic tendencies is still in its infancy. A handful of treatment modalities exist, but none is entirely satisfactory.

Immunotherapy (IT)

The basic principle of immunotherapy – also desensitization, or specific immunotherapy (SIT) – is to inject the sufferer with weak but increasingly strong doses of dilute allergen in order to 'persuade' an overreacting immune system to accept and tolerate exposure to the trigger. The doses are given weekly initially, and for a few months, and then at spaces of a month or two apart for up to four years. The conditions treated are presently limited principally to severe hay fever and dust-mite allergy.

Some patients do well on IT, and people allergic to birch pollen often find their cross-reactions to raw foods become milder.

On the negative side, the treatment is long, tedious, may not work, can trigger minor localized symptoms, and runs the risk of causing a more severe reaction.

Another form, called sub-lingual immunotherapy (SLIT), uses diluted drops of allergen under the tongue, and is popular in parts of continental Europe. Some trials using SLIT for food allergy have been promising.

Immunotherapy is not widely available, and is normally only offered to those whose quality of life is severely compromised by their illness. This may change, though, and further research may eventually yield an effective partial treatment for food allergies, so that a small accidental exposure may not result in a reaction.

Enzyme-potentiated desensitization (EPD)

This is a somewhat controversial form of desensitization which uses injections of dilute allergen in combination with an enzyme released by immune cells when they are stimulated. It is used for a wide range of sensitivities, including chemical intolerances, food allergies, asthma and food intolerances. Although there are some positive reports of benefits with EPD, equally there have been cases of unpleasant side effects. Orthodox medicine does not acknowledge its place in allergy treatment, and it is mostly only available privately.

Sodium cromoglycate (Nalcrom)

This is a non-steroidal anti-inflammatory drug, which acts as a mast-cell stabilizer, preventing the cells from releasing histamine in response to an allergen. However, it must be taken before exposure has taken place to have any effect.

It is mainly prescribed to people with asthma, who generally need to take the drug for some time in order to 'build up' its useful effects in the body. It can also be used on an as-needed basis: for instance, before exercise in those experiencing exercise-induced asthma.

Cromoglycate's use in food allergy is limited. It is used only exceptionally in patients with rapid-onset IgE reactions, largely because it does not always work. Its long-term usefulness is also unclear, and so it cannot come close to substituting permanent food avoidance, unfortunately.

That said, it is sometimes prescribed to those who have delayed IgE-mediated allergies, with symptoms such as eczema and urticaria in response to food, and infants and adults who react to a wide range of foods are sometimes helped by it.

Anti-IgE drugs

The development of drugs to disable IgE antibodies in the blood is one of the most exciting areas of research into the prevention of food-allergic reactions.

One, omalizumab (Xolair), has proved useful in allergic asthma and hay fever, but its potential for treating food allergies is less certain. Another, TNX-901, has shown greater promise in a small US-based study, where some peanut allergics after treatment were able to consume several peanuts without reacting. Trials with both have been subject to setbacks, and the drugs are expensive, so may not be widely available for some years.

Alternatives

Most so-called treatments available through alternative or fringe therapists are unproven and should be regarded with scepticism.

'Mind' therapies

Treatments like hypnotherapy and meditation may be of benefit to food-allergic patients, but only in the reduction of the anxiety associated with the condition. Some have suggested the severity of allergic responses can be reduced through such therapies, but objective studies are lacking.

Herbalism

Although some herbal remedies have been shown to have properties which can relieve asthma, eczema or hay fever, none is currently thought to have any use in food allergy, although this situation may change with further research.

Homoeopathy

This is based on the invented 'principle' that 'like cures like' – that a substance capable of producing a symptom can relieve that same symptom when administered heavily diluted or in minute doses. The British Society for Allergy and Clinical Immunology (BSACI) states that there is inadequate evidence for the efficacy of homoeopathic treatments in treating allergies, including food allergies. However, one or two respectable studies have shown minor possible benefits in hay fever sufferers.

Acupuncture

Although a proven treatment in pain relief and for mood elevation, acupuncture's role in treating symptoms of food allergy has not been validated. Some studies indicating that it may mildly relieve wheezing and hay fever are modestly encouraging. In Chinese medical practice, it would normally be used in conjunction with herbal treatments.

Nambudripad's Allergy Elimination Technique (NAET)

This is formulated on discredited diagnostic methods and Chinese principles of acupressure, and is increasingly popular in the USA and France. It is based on a flawed perception of allergy being caused by blockages of 'energy flow', which dismisses what is known about the immune system response. Dr Adrian Morris of the Surrey Allergy Clinic has dubbed NAET 'the most unsubstantiated allergy treatment proposed to date'.

Prevention

Our understanding of food allergies is not complete, and recommendations on how to prevent them in the unborn or the very young, or stop further ones developing in those already sensitized, should not be considered set in stone. Sadly, the research seems inconclusive in this area, and allergy experts are in occasional disagreement.

We know that inheritance is the most important factor in determining the likelihood of developing a predisposition towards allergy: if one parent is allergic, the likelihood is roughly one in three of a child being born with a tendency towards an allergy; if both are, the chance is around two in three.

However, other factors also come into play – such as diet, exposure to pets and dust, environmental conditions and overuse of antibiotics – and so divining the risks is subject to a wide margin of error, the study of allergy being an unpredictable science.

There may be, though, some steps you can take to reduce the odds.

Prevention during pregnancy

If you, your partner or another of your children is food-allergic, you will understandably be concerned about your unborn child.

The greatest worry is over peanut allergy. Department of Health guidelines, issued in the late nineties, put forward the suggestion that women from atopic families 'may wish' to avoid eating peanuts, in order to prevent any risk of their unborn baby being sensitized to allergenic proteins crossing the placental bloodstream – which some researchers believe may occur in the second half of pregnancy, not only to nut proteins, but to those in milk and egg too.

While this is possible, others have suggested it may be just as likely that an unborn child might develop *tolerance* towards an allergen if exposed to it *in utero*. Sadly, there is no conclusive study which demonstrates that avoidance in pregnancy has any preventative effect, making it difficult to offer conclusive advice to parents-to-be. Most professionals working in obstetrics and in allergy, however, will recommend you abstain from nuts and peanuts if allergies are a problem within your or your partner's immediate family.

If you are concerned about allergies to other foods, seek the advice of your allergist and perhaps a dietitian. Avoidance of milk in pregnancy, for instance, could compromise calcium intake, and should not be undertaken without professional supervision.

Avoiding active and passive smoking during pregnancy lessens the risk to your unborn child, and you should consume a varied and balanced diet, with adequate amounts of iron and folate, especially. Avoid alcohol, exposure to pollution and strong chemicals, and excessive contact with pets or house dust.

Take particular care to avoid any of your food allergens: the more reactions you have during pregnancy the more likely your child may inherit a disposition towards a similar allergy.

Prevention during breastfeeding

Once your child is born, if you can, breastfeed exclusively for at least four months, but preferably six, and try to continue non-exclusively beyond, as this may help prevent allergic development, particularly if there is a family history of the illness.

If breastfeeding is not possible, an extensively hydrolysed, or hydrolysate, formula feed may be recommended by your doctor or paediatric allergist. Hydrolysates are made from cow's milk, but because the proteins are mostly broken down into non-allergenic fragments, they are thought to reduce the risk of sensitization. They are not suitable for already sensitized babies, however, as some whole proteins may survive the hydrolysing process.

Amino-acid or elemental/hypoallergenic formulas such as Neocate are not made from cow's milk, and are considered extremely safe and effective for atopic babies.

The introduction of a non-hydrolysed cow's milk or cow's milk formula before six months, and especially before four months, should be avoided, as this is known to increase the risk of your baby developing a milk protein allergy. Further, according to Allergy UK: 'There is no place for soya formula or goat's milk formula in the primary prevention of allergy, as the susceptible baby is just as likely to become allergic to these as to cow's milk.'

It's generally accepted that breastfeeding babies can be sensitized through allergens consumed by the mother passing into her milk, and that this can occasionally bring on symptoms in infants too. If this is a concern, and you plan to avoid particular allergens while breastfeeding, speak to your consultant in the first instance. It is considered advisable to avoid peanuts and peanut-containing products during this time.

Again, protect your new baby from smoke and other allergens, but don't be paranoid about maintaining a scrupulously sterile environment in the home: too much cleanliness may have the opposite effect to that desired.

Prevention in infancy

Weaning should be delayed until at least four months, but preferably six. The introduction of solid foods should be done gradually, carefully and individually, under specialist guidance.

It's better to begin with cooked foods unlikely to trigger allergies, such as baby rice, pears, pureed root vegetables (carrot, sweet potatoes), green vegetables and, later, meats. Start with small amounts of one food, and gradually increase, before introducing another.

Once these have been incorporated, at between six and eight months, other foods can be given, such as grains (oats, wheat), pulses (peas, beans) and, very gradually, dairy-containing foods – although some endorse delaying the introduction of these even further.

Egg should not be introduced before one year; fish, later still.

Peanuts, tree nuts and shellfish should not be given to children younger than three – but some advise waiting until five.

If your baby is considered at risk of developing a particular allergy, you may like to further delay the introduction of that food. Also, always avoid introducing foods when a child is unwell.

With prepared foods, remember to read labels, and aim to give your child as pure a diet as possible, free from artificial colourings and preservatives. Check baby creams and nappy products too, for both food ingredients and additives.

These are only approximate guidelines, which can offer no guarantees. Different specialists hold different views, and research, which is inconclusive, is ongoing. Take up-to-date advice from your healthcare provider.

Is my infant developing a food allergy?

Closely monitor your baby through weaning for allergic symptoms. Consider keeping a food/symptom diary, which may be useful in identifying potential triggers to ill health and discomfort. Keep a daily record of everything you feed your child; especially make note of when new foods are introduced, and any symptoms.

Signs to watch out for include:

- urticaria, skin blotches, eczema;
- swelling anywhere on the body;
- colic, vomiting, diarrhoea, constipation, abnormal stools;
- persistant rhinitis or nasal symptoms;
- regular wheezing or coughing;
- ear infections, discharge or discomfort;
- refusing to breastfeed, food rejection or obvious problems eating;
- any other unusual symptoms or unexplained changes in behaviour.

If symptoms present themselves, see your doctor or paediatrician promptly.

Prevention in childhood and adulthood

There is little research on preventing new or additional food allergies developing beyond infancy, and again it is difficult to give firm advice.

Maintaining a good, varied diet can only benefit your health, so ensure yours is up to scratch. Avoiding tobacco, alcohol and unnecessary drugs and medicines is also likely to help, as is reducing your exposure to other allergens. If you work in food processing, ensure you are protected with overalls, gloves and face masks where practical.

Gut integrity

Most of the mooted ideas in allergy prevention centre on maintaining a healthy digestive system.

An adequate intake of probiotics and prebiotics (see p. 82) may help people of all ages, according to several Scandinavian studies, although the mechanisms are not yet understood.

Some studies have suggested that a diet rich in omega 3s (found in oily fish, linseed, walnuts, hemp seeds and soya beans) can help reduce the production of allergy antibodies, and it is known that essential fatty acids help the gut membranes.

Abnormally high gut permeability – dubbed 'leaky gut syndrome' (LGS) – is another possible cause of greater susceptibility to food allergies. In LGS, the gut wall, which usually allows only small digested food molecules to pass through it into the bloodstream, becomes inflamed or irritated, allowing larger, undigested protein molecules to enter, possibly sensitizing the individual or triggering an immune response. Some have suggested that by preventing LGS, atopic individuals may reduce their risks of developing further allergies.

Factors which may contribute to LGS, and which therefore may be worth avoiding where possible, include:

- medicines, painkillers and drugs;
- alcohol, tobacco and excessive caffeine;
- refined sugar, processed foods, food additives;
- spicy foods (chilli, hot curry);
- enzymic fruits (papaya, mango, pineapple) on an empty stomach;
- chronic stress;
- environmental toxins;
- food poisoning.

It is worth getting any sporadic or chronic digestive malaises you suffer from – such as IBS, indigestion, heartburn – investigated and resolved, as their underlying causes may in some cases make you also more susceptible to allergies and food intolerances. One interesting study from Austria found that antacid or indigestion pills made food-allergic reactions more likely, possibly because they interfere with the breakdown and neutralization of potentially allergenic proteins in the digestive system. As so often is the case in medicine, it may be better to investigate and cure the root cause, rather than merely treat or mask any symptoms you're experiencing.

Maintaining good eating habits is highly recommended: don't skip meals, don't eat on the go, do eat slowly and deliberately, don't overeat in one sitting, don't drink too much alcohol or acidic fluids (wine, orange juice) with your meals, and always avoid fad diets.

These subjects are explored more fully in this book's companion title, *Living with Food Intolerance* (Sheldon, 2005).

Conclusion

The outlook

Life for food allergics in the twenty-first century is infinitely preferable to that 15 or even 10 years ago, when food allergies were rarer, not widely recognized or well understood, and little support or advice was available.

Now, those working in the food industry are increasingly understanding of those on restricted diets, manufacturers are catering extensively for them, and food labelling is getting better – although room for improvement remains. The Government is slowly waking up to the allergy epidemic, and healthcare provision is likely to advance in the UK over coming years, thanks in large part to the committed lobbying of the allergy charities. Cautious optimism about several drugs being looked at in the USA is certainly justified.

Research projects should soon come to fruition. EuroPrevall is a four-year EU-funded project co-ordinated by the Institute of Food Research. Scientists are carrying out epidemiological studies, and hope to determine the role of diet, environment and infections in the development of food allergy, to formulate more precise diagnostic methods, catalogue all known allergens and their chemical idiosyncrasies, and help predict potential cross-reacting foods. Economic costs and quality-of-life impact of allergic illness will also be looked at. EuroPrevall's overarching mission is to improve life for food allergics. You can keep updated at www.europrevall.org.

Other pieces of research may eventually contribute to the larger food allergy puzzle, bringing a clearer picture into focus. Finnish researchers have been looking at the value of probiotic supplementation, for instance, while Japanese scientists have isolated a compound in green tea which appears to block IgE and histamine production, at least *in vitro*.

Genetically modified (GM) food and crop science offer tantalizing possibilities. So-called allergy-free GM nuts have been produced, and selecting and nurturing strains of food which lack particular allergenic proteins is another path being explored – in Sweden, for instance, a country with a severe birch pollen–apple syndrome problem, cultivating low-allergen apple breeds is under investigation.

Perhaps less obviously appealing but potentially more remarkable is research into the role parasitic worms play in allergy prevention. This works on the premise that immune systems are kept too preoccupied with internal parasites to 'bother' reacting to allergens. If a chemical or biological trigger can be isolated and harnessed, a cure could be developed in the future . . . hopefully without needing to infect people with wriggly guests.

Less positively, we know that food allergies are on the increase, and whether healthcare can keep up with demand is a moot point. There are alarming signs that allergies to carbohydrate components are emerging, and some researchers expect to see new allergies to foods whose popularity is predicted to rise – such as caraway, linseed and hemp.

Overall though, the positives without question outweigh the negatives.

What can I do to help?

Read relevant publications such as *Foods Matter* and *Allergy*, understand the key issues, and keep abreast of what is happening in the world of food allergy – not only for your own benefit, but also in order to accurately 'spread the word' to others. At a time when some of the loudest commentators on sensitivities include svelte celebrities claiming weight loss following purported allergy diagnoses, it is vital to get grounded messages across.

Recommend good products or services to relevant people. Challenge and report shoddy service or carelessly labelled goods. If allergy provision in your part of the country is dismal, report it to your MP.

Finally, become an active member and supporter of charities such as the Anaphylaxis Campaign, Allergy UK and Action Against Allergy. Theirs are tireless endeavours, and the more of us who can participate and share in their goals, the more likely the food allergy epidemic will one day be beaten, to the benefit of all.

Appendix 1: tests and diagnoses

If you have been experiencing symptoms of food allergy, a full evaluation is warranted. Your doctor may refer you to an allergy consultant or clinic for professional assessment, although because of a dearth of allergy provision on the NHS, this may be some distance from your home, and only after several months.

However, some doctors have only a sketchy understanding of food allergy, and may mistakenly believe you to be suffering from another condition. If you are dissatisfied with your doctor's assessment, private medicine may be an option. The allergy charities can advise on reputable consultants. NHS and private clinics are listed at www.specialistinfo.com. BUPA is on 0800 600 500; www.bupa.co.uk.

Food-allergy diagnosis

Diagnosis of food allergy can only be made with any degree of confidence by a trained clinical doctor or allergist using a process combining an holistic assessment of you, the patient, with a consideration of your symptoms, and your medical and family history, and good – but by no means infallible – laboratory and out-patient testing procedures. In some cases, you may be asked to submit to a food challenge.

Other past or present allergic conditions, such as asthma or pollen sensitivity, must be considered, as must seasonal or environmental sensitivities or reactions, possible occupational exposure to food products, and other reactions to foods, such as intolerances. Physical tests of lung functioning, and examinations of the eyes, nose and skin, can help your specialist determine which, if any, tests you should undergo.

Skin prick testing (SPT)

SPT involves placing a drop of diluted allergen onto the skin of your forearm, then piercing the skin through the drop with a tiny needle. Itching within minutes, and the development of a swollen red weal at the site, are indicative of a positive reaction – the larger the weal, the stronger the response. Because such a minuscule amount of allergen is used, SPT is extremely safe; the odds of anaphylaxis resulting from it run into the millions.

A positive response to a food allergen only sometimes means you are allergic to it. You may have a positive SPT to an allergen which causes no reaction in the context of everyday exposure, or even to an allergen to which you reacted as a child, but have since outgrown.

A negative response is more valuable diagnostically, as it usually signifies you are not allergic. False negatives can occur, however, if your reaction is weak or delayed, you are taking antihistamines, or in the case of fruit or vegetables, some of whose allergens are unstable.

The accuracy of a positive SPT is around 55 per cent; with a negative, it is 95 per cent+. Some allergens, such as soya or apple, produce less reliable results; others, like fish and nuts, are more trustworthy.

SPT is suitable for all ages, and can be a useful adjunct to diagnosis.

Blood testing

Various tests may be used to ascertain IgE levels to individual allergens present in your blood, including RAST and CAP.

Negative results are fairly reliable (around 90 per cent), though false negatives are possible, especially if you have already excluded the suspect from your diet. Positive blood tests have a reliability of just above 50 per cent, and can only contribute towards or help confirm a diagnosis, but never provide one exclusively of other tests or factors. Equally, they cannot generally give a reliable indication of the severity of any possible allergy.

Home blood testing

Some home testing kits for IgE antibodies are available from private laboratories or pharmacists. A few provide immediate positive or negative results to a specific allergen; others require you to return a drop of blood for analysis.

While many of these are clinically sound in principle, a diagnosis reached on the basis of such a test in the absence of a professional medical consultation is ill-advised. Blood analyses can only ever form one piece of the allergy puzzle, therefore home testing cannot be recommended, at least certainly not in isolation.

Exclusion diet

Often called an elimination diet, this is a diagnostic diet which aims to remove the suspect foods from your diet for a period of, say, a fortnight, or until symptoms disappear, and then introduce foods individually to see whether they return.

It is rarely used in allergy diagnosis, and only then when delayed and non-life threatening symptoms, such as eczema, are experienced. It is more common in the diagnosis of food intolerance, when it may be used by both dietitians and allergists.

Challenge testing

A food allergy can be indicated if symptoms manifest when you are challenged with the food, especially after you have previously eliminated it from your diet.

Open challenging means you're aware of what you're being challenged with, and is not reliable; single blind challenging means the tester is aware and you are not; and double blind challenging – considered the 'gold standard' – means neither of you are aware, removing all bias.

Challenge testing is time-consuming, costly, often risky, and it can be difficult to effectively disguise the appearance, taste and texture of foods in blind testing. As there is no universally accepted protocol on precisely how challenges ought to be administered, various techniques and systems have sprung up.

A once popular procedure was to offer food disguised within a gelatine capsule, though this has fallen out of favour as it bypasses the oral mucosal membranes. Occasionally, the food may be 'hidden' within another, such as a broth or a biscuit. However, this 'masking' may not provide an accurate reflection of how a food may normally be consumed, and so some testers have concluded that it's better to give the food being tested in a form in which the patient would expect to encounter it in practice.

Typically, exposure is gradual at first, with perhaps a small dose being applied to your skin or lip, and then into the mouth, and then by ingestion of increasing amounts. Each stage is separated by at least ten minutes, while any possible reactions are carefully monitored.

If the challenge is positive at any stage, a positive diagnosis can be confidently made.

In the event of a negative challenge, a larger portion of the food may be openly given to confirm the diagnosis and offer reassurance. A good clinic will often 'chase' a negative diagnosis, to ensure that the patient has reincorporated the suspect food back into their diet, and is not suffering adverse effects.

Food challenges cannot usually be performed on those who have asthma or who may be at risk of anaphylaxis. They are only undertaken under close scrutiny, with resuscitation equipment and medication at hand.

Forms of challenge testing can also be useful when a patient suspects that an allergy may have been outgrown, wishes to reintroduce a doubtful food, or would like to check the safety of a potential cross-reactor, or even the cooked or raw versions of the food, when a reaction to only one is confirmed.

When multiple allergens are suspected, it may be useful for patients to be put on an exclusion diet prior to challenge testing.

OAS diagnosis

Diagnosis of hay fever is typically made through circumstantial and symptomatic evidence: if you experience severe rhinitis and conjunctivitis during summer months, for example, a doctor may confidently suspect you have grass-pollen hay fever. Where there is doubt, SPTs for specific pollens may be performed, and these can help indicate potential cross-reacting foods.

These fruits and vegetables may also be tested for, but because the allergens associated with OAS are prone to degradation, fresh rather than stored sample extracts produce more reliable results, and many allergists are increasingly using them, adopting a modified SPT technique called Prick plus Prick testing (or Scratch plus Scratch). Here, the test food is first pricked, and then the patient's forearm is pricked, thereby introducing into the epidermis a fresh extract gathered on the tip of the lancet.

Latex–food cross-reactions

Latex allergy can be diagnosed effectively through blood testing, but similar testing for associated food allergies appears to be poor at indicating triggers. In one study, only a third of latex allergics reporting symptoms to cross-reacting fruits tested blood positive to those fruits.

Alternative tests

Poor NHS allergy provision and long waiting lists for assessment have conspired to create a gaping diagnostic vacuum in the UK which alternative therapists, touting a number of food sensitivity tests of deeply suspect value, are gladly filling.

Practitioners can be extremely persuasive. You may be told that orthodox diagnostic techniques are not foolproof – something the medical profession freely acknowledges – or that doctors are dismissive of food allergy and unsympathetic of its sufferers – an unfair and sweeping generalization.

Another complicating factor is that some therapists adopt vague or inaccurate definitions of both food allergy and food intolerance, and don't always draw an agreed distinction between the two, leaving the patient confused as to what, exactly, is purportedly being tested for.

Some of the tests available include:

- applied kinesiology, where samples of the tested food are placed under the tongue or in the hand, and the arm muscles are tested for strength – a weakened response being supposedly indicative of sensitivity;
- electrodermal skin-testing techniques – including Vega, BEST, Dermatron, Listen and Quantum – which look for changes in skin resistance in response to allergens held within an electrical circuit;
- hair or fingernail analysis, which looks for assorted mineral traces, from which conclusions about food sensitivities are drawn;
- cytotoxicity testing – a technique of adding allergens to the patient's blood cells in a test tube, and monitoring responses to reach deductions about sensitivity.

Results follow a strikingly similar pattern. One or both of wheat or dairy are commonly cited as culprits, and to these will be added other supposed allergens, often including obscure foods (broad bean appears a favourite), in order to lend the whole operation a convincing air of precision. In fact, multiple and unrelated food allergies are comparatively rare, and the restricted diets demanded by the results of such tests can put you at risk of under-nutrition. Equally, a false-negative result to a particular food can constitute unreliable and unsafe reassurance that you are not allergic to a possible trigger.

None of these tests is reliable, then. All are either clinically unproven or have been discredited by independent medical studies – facts which, incidentally, the practitioner is unlikely to disclose to you.

If you are prepared to pay for private testing, ask your doctor or the allergy charities for a reputable private clinic or hospital which can undertake skin prick, blood or challenge testing, and be wary of natural health or Chinese herbal medicine stores bearing 'Allergy Testing Here' signs on their windows.

Appendix 2: food families

Cross-reactions often occur between related foods. The following can give an indication of those you might need to avoid should you be allergic to one or more family members.

Plant foods

Any not categorized below are likely to form one-member groups, with no common close edible relatives – examples include amaranth, bananas (including plantains), capers, coffee, elderberry, linseed, ginkgo biloba, ginseng, grapes, kiwi, lychee, olives, papaya, peppercorns, persimmon, pineapple, poppy seed, sesame, sweet potato, tea and vanilla, as well as many of the tree nuts. However, being an 'only child' is not predictive of a food's reactive potential – kiwis are highly allergenic, for instance, while tea is not.

Besides, cross-reactions are also possible between unrelated foods. The tree nuts are a case in point. Although many are individualists, they often cross-react with one another, and with peanut, a legume, and almond, a rose member. It's a similar picture with many seeds.

For an exceptionally thorough taxonomic guide to both common and obscure culinary and medicinal plants, see www.purr.demon. co.uk/Food/RelatedPlantList.html, compiled by researcher Jack Campin and food-allergy dietitian Marion Bowles. The list is in English and Latin, helpful for identifying ingredients in non-food products too.

Carrot family: angelica, aniseed, caraway, carrot, celeriac, celery, chervil, coriander, cumin, dill, fennel, lovage, parsley, parsnip.
Citrus family: bergamot, grapefruit, lemon, lime, kumquat, orange, tangerine, and hybrids such as clementine and ugli.
Daisy family: artichoke (globe and Jerusalem), burdock, camomile, cardoon, chicory, dandelion, echinacea, endive, feverfew, lettuce, milk thistle, salsify, safflower, sunflower, tarragon.
Goosefoot family: beetroot, chard, spinach, sugar beet; also, but more distantly, quinoa.

Grass family: a large family providing many edible grains. As far as cross-reactions go, the following sub-families are more relevant:

- barley, kamut, rye, spelt, triticale, wheat; also, but more distantly, oats (all are gluten grains);
- maize, millet, sorghum, sweetcorn;
- rice, wild rice.

Legume family: alfalfa, beans (such as broad, butter, haricot, kidney, mung, runner, soya – but not cocoa), carob (locust bean), chickpea, fenugreek, lentil, liquorice, lupin, mangetout, pea, peanut, tamarind – and any edible sprouts, such as beansprouts or peanut shoots. Also, legumes used to make additive gums or supplements – acacia, clover, guar, senna, tara, tragacanth.

Lily family: aloe vera, asparagus, chives, garlic, leek, onion, shallot, spring onion.

Melon family: cucumber, courgette, marrow, melon (all varieties, including honeydew and watermelon), pumpkin, squash.

Mustard family: broccoli, Brussels sprouts, cabbages, cauliflower, Chinese leaf, collard greens, cress, horseradish, kale, kohlrabi, mustard, pak choi, radish, rape (canola), rocket, swede (rutabaga), turnip, watercress.

Nightshade family: peppers (capsicum and chilli, as well as paprika), physalis (Cape gooseberry), potato, tomato; also aubergine, but cross-reactions with it seem rare.

Rose family: a large family that gives us many fruits. With regard to cross-reactions, these subdivisions are more pertinent:

- apricot, cherry, damson, greengage, nectarine, peach, plum/prune, sloe – also almond;
- apple and pear;
- strawberry;
- blackberry, boysenberry, loganberry, raspberry.

Other families

All the above families appear to be the most relevant in food-allergic reactions, especially when sensitivity to pollen is involved. The following appear less so, and their members may be less likely to cross-react. This is especially true when different parts of the plants are used as food – as with the laurels, where fruits (avocado), leaves (bay) and bark (cinnamon) are consumed.

- cashew family (cashew, mango, pistachio);
- currant family (blackcurrant, gooseberry, redcurrant);
- dead-nettle family (basil, lavender, mint, marjoram, oregano, rosemary, sage, thyme);
- ginger family (cardamom, ginger, turmeric);
- knotweed family (buckwheat, rhubarb, sorrel);
- laurel family (avocado, bay, camphor, cinnamon);
- mulberry family (breadfruit, fig, mulberry);
- myrtle family (allspice, clove, eucalyptus, guava);
- palm family (coconut, date, palm, saw palmetto).

Seafood

These divide into three distinct categories – fish, crustaceans and molluscs – the first and third being sub-divided further.

In general, the closer related any two sea animals are, the more likely you will experience cross-reactions between them – in the case of fish, cross-reactions between bony fish and cartilagenous fish are the least likely.

Crustaceans and molluscs are often grouped together colloquially as 'shellfish'. There is some evidence that the likelihood of cross-reactions between these two groups is higher than that between either group and fish.

Fish

Cartilagenous fish form one class – members are monkfish, ray, shark and skate.

Bony fish form a numerically dominant class, and can be divided into a number of orders, of which the following are the most important:

- clupeiformes – anchovy, herring, pilchard/sardine, sprat;
- gadiformes – cod, haddock, hake, whiting;
- perciformes – bass, bream, mackerel, perch, red mullet, snapper, swordfish, tuna, yellowtail;

111

- pleuronectiformes – flounder, halibut, plaice, sole, turbot;
- salmoniformes – pike, salmon, trout, whitefish.

Crustaceans

- Crab, crayfish, langouste, lobster, prawn, shrimp.

Molluscs

- bivalves – clam, cockle, mussel, oyster, scallop, whelk;
- cephalopods – cuttlefish, octopus, squid;
- gastropods – abalone, limpet, periwinkle, snail.

Useful addresses

Support organizations

Allergy UK
3 White Oak Square
London Road
Swanley
Kent BR8 7AG
Allergy Helpline: 01322 619898
Website: www.allergyuk.org

The Anaphylaxis Campaign
PO Box 275
Farnborough
Hampshire GU14 6SX
Tel.: 01252 373793
Helpline: 01252 542029
Website: www.anaphylaxis.org.uk

Action Against Allergy
PO Box 278
Twickenham
Middlesex TW1 4QQ
Tel.: 020 8892 2711
Website: www.actionagainstallergy.co.uk
Email: AAA@actionagainstallergy.freeserve.co.uk

Asthma UK
Summit House
70 Wilson Street
London EC2A 2DB
Tel.: 020 7786 4900
Advice line: 08457 01 02 03
Website: www.asthma.org.uk

Latex Allergy Support Group
PO Box 27
Filey
YO14 9YH
Helpline: 07071 225838 (7–10 pm, Monday to Friday)
Website: www.lasg.co.uk

Websites

foodallergens.ifr.ac.uk
The Institute of Food Research's food allergens database. Complex, but useful to those experiencing idiosyncratic reactions, who need to be aware of other potential triggers.

housedustmite.org
Advice on controlling and managing dust mite allergy.

www.allallergy.net
A portal to hundreds of organisations, events, publications and products worldwide.

www.allergy-network.co.uk and www.allergy-clinic.co.uk
Excellent sites by Dr Adrian Morris of the Surrey Allergy Clinic.

www.allergy.org.au
Australian Society of Clinical Immunology and Allergy (ASCIA).

www.allergyinschools.co.uk
Aimed at helping children with life-threatening allergies; includes information for teachers and school caterers.

www.allergysa.org
Allergy Society of South Africa.

www.bsaci.org
British Society for Allergy and Clinical Immunology.

www.eatwell.gov.uk
Foods Standard Agency-run site with advice on food safety, food labelling and more.

www.eczema.org
The National Eczema Society.

www.faia.org.uk
The Food Additives and Ingredients Association.

www.foodallergy.org
The Food Allergy & Anaphylaxis Network (USA).

www.foodallergyinitiative.org
Excellent US resource filled with information, news and research.

www.foodyoucaneat.com
Recipes and other resources for food-allergic people (USA).

www.nonuts.co.uk
Very useful site for nut-allergics, rich in consumer information.

www.pollenuk.co.uk
National Pollen and Aerobiology Research Unit.

www.sojasun.com
Producers of soya-based probiotic drinks.

www.tauk.org
Teen Allergy UK – a forum for older children and young adults.

www.vegansociety.com
The Vegan Society. Advice on fish-, dairy- and egg-free living.

www.vegsoc.org
The Vegetarian Society. Advice on fish-free eating.

www.worldallergy.org
The World Allergy Organization.

www.yorktest.com
Specialists in food intolerance testing in laboratories in York; they
also offer multi-allergy (food and inhalants) testing.

Online discussion/support groups

Web-based forums can offer terrific support and information, though some can be unruly at times. Advice is generally well meant, but can never replace authoritative medical opinion. Many are US-based, so be aware of differences in definitions, healthcare systems and labelling, for instance. Here are four, but you can find others through some of the resources above, or try a search ('food allergy discussion' or 'allergy forum', for instance).

groups.google.com/group/alt.support.food-allergies
A lively forum for food allergics and their carers.

groups.yahoo.com/group/foodallergykitchen
Forum dedicated to allergen-free recipes and cooking.

health.groups.yahoo.com/group/fasters/
'Food Allergy Survivors Together' – a friendly, fun, supportive group for sufferers and loved ones.

health.groups.yahoo.com/group/FCMYI
'Food Can Make You Ill' – a group open to those suffering from food sensitivities, their relatives, and interested professionals.

Events

The Allergy Show – www.allergyshow.co.uk
An annual consumer event covering all allergies, food included, with hundreds of exhibitors. It's held in June at Olympia, London.

Retailers and manufacturers

Supermarkets

Most supermarkets and larger stores stock ranges of special-diet foods, both their own brands and other manufacturers' as well. Many produce 'free from' leaflets detailing these and other products, with a breakdown of ingredients, which can be mailed to you, while some offer information on their websites or answer questions via email.

The customer service numbers listed are manned by staff who can advise.

Asda. 0500 100055; www.asda.co.uk
Boots. 0845 070 8090; www.boots.com
Budgens. 0800 526002; www.budgens.co.uk
Co-op. 0800 068 6727; www.co-op.co.uk.
Iceland. 01244 842842; www.iceland.co.uk
Kwik Save. 0117 935 6669; www.kwiksave.co.uk
Marks & Spencer. 0845 302 1234; www.marksandspencer.com
Morrisons. 01924 870000; www.morrisons.co.uk
J Sainsbury. 0800 636262; www.sainsburys.co.uk
Somerfield. 0117 935 6669; www.somerfield.co.uk
Tesco. 0800 505555; www.tesco.com
Waitrose. 0800 188884; www.waitrose.com

Health food stores

Both the national chains and your smaller local stores are likely to be good sources of products free from wheat, dairy, eggs, soya, fish and other allergens.

Holland and Barrett. 0870 606 6605; www.hollandandbarrett.co.uk

GNC. 0845 601 3248; www.gnc.co.uk

Mail order and on-line suppliers

Allergy Free Direct. 01288 356396; www.allergyfreedirect.com
A wide range of specialist foods free from yeast, wheat, dairy, egg and tomato.

GoodnessDirect. 0871 871 6611; www.goodnessdirect.co.uk
Three thousand products free from wheat, dairy, egg and yeast; vegan/vegetarian foods too.

Wheatanddairyfree.com
Several hundred products free from wheat, dairy, yeast and egg.

'Free-from' food companies and suppliers

Alpro. 0800 018 8180; www.alprosoya.co.uk
Soya-based milks, creams, yogurts and desserts.

Bakers Delight. 0845 120 0038; www.bakers-delight.co.uk

Wheat- and gluten-free bread, cakes, pies and puddings.

Clearspring Ltd. 020 8749 1781; www.clearspring.co.uk
Guaranteed nut-free seed snacks (e.g. pumpkin and sunflower) and other dairy-, egg- and wheat-free specialist foods.

Community Foods Ltd, agents for Orgran. 020 8208 2966; www.orgran.com
Snacks, cereals and pastas free of wheat, dairy and egg.

D&D. 024 7637 0909; www.d-dchocolates.com
Carob and dairy-free/gluten-free chocolate bars and seasonal products.

DariFree. 01908 200365; www.darifree.co.uk
Potato milk and associated products.

Doves Farm. 01488 684880; www.dovesfarm.co.uk
Cereals and baked goods free from wheat and other allergens.

Fabulous Bakin' Boys. 01993 777444; www.bakinboys.co.uk
Nut-free flapjacks, muffins, biscuits and other treats.

Fayrefield Foods. 01270 589311; www.fayrefield.com
Swedish Glacé dairy-free ice cream and cholesterol-lowering milk.

First Foods. 01494 431355; www.first-foods.com
Dairy- and soya-free oat milk, cream, ice cream and choc ices.

Green's. 0113 250 2036; www.glutenfreebeers.co.uk
Gluten-free/wheat-free beers.

Gluten Free Foods. 020 8953 4444; www.glutenfree-foods.co.uk
Producers of the Glutano, Barkat, Tritamyl and Valpiform gluten-free ranges.

Hambleton Ales. 01765 640108; www.hambletonales.co.uk
Gluten-free/wheat-free beers.

It's Nut Free Ltd. 01765 641890; www.itsnutfree.com
Guaranteed nut-free chocolate, birthday cakes, biscuits, Christmas puddings and other treats.

Heron Quality Foods. +353 (0)23 39006; www.glutenfreedirect.com
Irish co-operative producing wheat-free foods.

Kallo Foods. 01428 685100; www.kallofoods.com
Dairy-free rice milk, and wheat-free crackers, biscuits and bread-sticks.

Kinnerton. 020 7284 9500; www.kinnerton.com
Guaranteed nut-free chocolate confectionery, including Easter and Christmas lines.

Matthew Foods Ltd. 0800 028 4499; www.purespreads.com
Dairy-free spreads.

MH Foods. 01322 337711; www.mh-foods.co.uk
Fish-free Worcestershire sauce, dairy-free Parmazano (Parmesan cheese replacement), egg-free mayonnaise and other nut-free, wheat-free and vegan products.

Nutricia. 01225 711801; www.glutafin.co.uk/www.trufree.co.uk
Gluten- and wheat-free ranges of bread, biscuits and pasta.

Nutrition Point. 07041 544044; www.nutritionpoint.co.uk
Dietary Specials range of wheat-free breads, biscuits, cake mixes, pasta products, ready meals.

Organico RealFoods. 01189 238760; www.organico.co.uk
Hazelnut, almond and quinoa 'milks'.

Orgran. See Community Foods Ltd.

Plamil Foods. 01303 854207; www.plamilfoods.co.uk
Non-dairy milks, chocolate and drinks, and egg-free mayonnaises.

Redwood Foods. 01536 400557; www.redwoodfoods.co.uk

Soya-based Cheezly dairy-free cheese replacements and fish-free 'fishcakes' and 'fish fingers'.

Scheese. 01700 505357; www.scheese.co.uk
Soya-based 'cheeses'.

So Good. 0800 328 0423; www.sogood123.com
Soya milks.

Soma Organics. 0870 950 7662; www.somafoods.com
'Nomato' tomato-free range of baked beans, ketchup, soup, chilli and pasta sauce.

Tiger White Drinks. www.tigerwhitedrinks.com
Tiger White dairy-free sedge-root/chufa milk.

Triano Foods. 020 8861 4443; www.trianobrands.co.uk
Dairy-free desserts (Tofutti), cream 'cheeses' and fish pâtés.

The Village Bakery. 01768 881811; www.village-bakery.com/
www.ok-foods.co.uk
Wheat- and dairy-free cakes, puddings, biscuits and fruit bars.

Other suppliers

Advanced Allergy Technologies. 0161 998 1999;
www.allergy.uk.com
Anti-allergen filters, bedding, respiratory masks and clothing.

ALK-Abelló. 01488 686016; www.epipen.co.uk and
www.alk-abello.co.uk
Distributors of the EpiPen. Website offers information on usage and allergy management. Register to receive newsletters, offers and alerts.

Allergy Matters. 020 8339 0029/0800 052 8228;
www.allergymatters.com
A 'one-stop allergy shop' selling products for all allergic conditions.

Dietarycard. 01506 635358; www.dietarycard.co.uk

Personalised food alert cards for use in hotels and restaurants in the UK and abroad, with translations available in several languages to help articulate specific needs.

Hoopers. 0121 200 1616; www.hoopers.org/Mediset.htm
Jewellery (necklaces, bracelets, watches) to alert medical staff to allergies.

The Insurance Surgery. 0800 083 2829;
www.the-insurance-surgery.co.uk
Health and life insurance and financial services advice aimed at allergy sufferers.

Lincoln Medical. 01722 410443; www.anapen.co.uk
Distributor of the Anapen.

MedicAlert. 020 7833 3034/0800 581420;
www.medicalert.org.uk (UK) and www.medicalert.org (international)
Charity providing identification bracelets and necklets (Emblems), supported by a 24-hour emergency telephone service in over 100 languages.

Medicare Plus. 01737 226384; www.medicareplus.co.uk
Allergy medication carrying-cases.

Select Wisely. (+00 1) 973 729 6538; www.selectwisely.com
Translation cards.

The Yellow Cross Company. 01252 820321;
www.yellowcross.co.uk
Sturdy travelling bags and containers for adrenaline pens, asthma inhalers and antihistamine syrups, as well as translation cards (including Asian languages).

Further reading

Books and publications

Committee on Toxicity of Chemicals in Food, Consumer Products and the Environment, *Adverse Reactions to Food and Food Ingredients*. FSA, London, 2000.

Gamlin, Linda, *The Allergy Bible*. Quadrille, London, 2005.

Gazzola, Alex, *Living with Food Intolerance*. Sheldon Press, London, 2005.

Koeller, Kim, and La France, Robert, *Let's Eat Out! Your Passport to Living Gluten and Allergy Free*. R&R Publishing, Chicago, 2005.

McGee, Paul, *SUMO. Shut Up, Move On: The Straight-Talking Guide to Creating and Enjoying a Brilliant Life*. Capstone Publishing Ltd, Oxford, 2005.

Royal College of Physicians, *Allergy: The Unmet Need*. RCP, London, 2003.

Statham, Bill, *The Chemical Maze: Your Guide to Food Additives and Cosmetic Ingredients*. Summersdale, Chichester, 2006.

Ursell, Amanda, *L is for Labels*. Hay House, London, 2004.

Wright, Tanya, *Food Allergies*. Class Publishing, London, 2006.

Youngson, Dr Robert, *Coping Successfully with Hay Fever*. Sheldon Press, London, 1995.

Magazines

Foods Matter magazine
5 Lawn Road
London NW3 2XS
Tel.: 020 7722 2866
Website: www.foodsmatter.com
Email: info@foodsmatter.com

Allergy magazine
PSP Communications
13–15 Craven Street
London WC2N 5AD
Tel.: 020 7747 9390
Website: www.allergymagazine.com
Email: allergy@pspcom.com

Living Without magazine
PO Box 2126
Northbrook
IL 60065, USA
Tel.: 00 1 847 480 8810
Website: www.LivingWithout.com
Email: editor@LivingWithout.com

Allergic Living magazine
2100 Bloor Street West, Suite 6-168,
Toronto
Ontario M6S 5A5, Canada
Tel.: 00 1 888 771 7747
Website: www.allergicliving.com
Email: info@allergicliving.com

Index